INTERNAL CLEANSING
is an
OLD MOVEMENT

INTERNAL CLEANSING
is an
OLD MOVEMENT

by Lee DuBelle

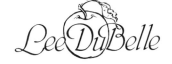

ISBN: 0-9618703-2-X

Cover, Page Design and Illustrations
   by Roberta Sinnock, Tucson, Arizona
Typography and Book Production
   by Walsh and Associates, Tempe, Arizona

Printed in the United States of America

Dedication

To my
adopted mother,
Louise.

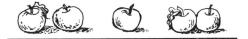

Acknowledgement

I would like to acknowledge the
help given to me by Rosemary, Roberta
and Ken without whom this book might
never have been published.
My thanks also to Althea, Val Jean,
Barbara, and Anne for their time and
interest in the project. Each contributed
constructive suggestions which helped
me understand the public's need.

Table of Contents

Illustrations

Introduction

Over the past 25 to 30 years, Lee DuBelle has researched the ideas outlined in this book, using the most responsive testing equipment available: her own body and its health and well being.

The result is a system of internal cleansing that produces dynamic health, effective digestion and a high level of energy. By eliminating toxins from the body, we avoid a wide range of maladies and illnesses and reverse the harm we have done to our bodies through years of improper eating.

To see Lee DuBelle today, one would never believe that at one time in her life she suffered from obesity, mental and physical exhaustion, tuberculosis spots on her lungs, extremely low blood pressure, pre-menstrual syndrome, cysts on one ovary, bleeding stomach ulcers and a prolapsed colon. She also smoked three packs of cigarettes a day. Using the food combining and internal cleansing techniques she discovered herself, she has stopped smoking and overcome her physical ailments. In addition, she has tremendous energy which allows her to travel the nation giving lectures and seminars on Proper Food Combining, Internal Cleansing, and other related topics.

Internal Cleansing is an Old Movement is the result of years of continuing personal research and consultations with clients on nearly every physical difficulty imaginable.

Ken Bacher

CHAPTER ONE

Why Internal Cleansing Is Necessary

Suppose someone told you that you need some fat or oil to keep your skin healthy. So you decide you'll rub fat all over your body.

Then they say you need lots of protein, so you rub protein all over your body.

Then they tell you that you need some carbohydrates, so you rub some carbohydrates on your body. You keep doing this for 20 years. Once in a while you wash off with a little splatter of water, never really washing thoroughly, just a little rinsing.

What do you think the condition of your skin would be at the end of that 20 years? One thing you know is that it would be a little bit thicker. You wouldn't smell too good, either; in fact, you'd probably downright stink. And you would probably weigh more. Now suppose that finally, after 20 years, you decide, "Well, I've had it." So you start washing and scraping it off. Do you know that in that length of time, you may have accumulated 10 to 20 pounds of garbage? Maybe even 30 to 40!

Underneath all those pounds of garbage there may be sores and lesions and other things that you had no idea would be there. In fact, it could be so bad that the tissue could be rotting. That is exactly what's been going on inside of us for years and years.

People's bodies are full of old layers of fats, starch and proteins in the form of feces, mucus, gases and toxins. Due to years of this accumulation, their insides are a little bit thicker, they weigh more, and they downright stink. They have internal sores and the tissue is starting to rot.

Millions of people have spent billions of dollars on soaps, cleansers, perfumes, oils, creams, body brushes, and so forth, to make sure the outside of their body looks, feels and smells good. Millions of hours have been spent learning about the skin and how to care for it; and many books are available to teach you about the outside of your body.

However, most of these same people know very little about the inside of their bodies. The main cleansing you need is on the *inside* and if that is clean, it will reflect on the *outside*.

We've all heard the saying, "True beauty comes from within." Well, that's what I say about health. True health comes from within. That can only happen when your "internal cleansing is an old movement."

When people start internal cleansing, they notice things about their body that they never before had even imagined. They notice relief from old aches and pains. Sometimes with cleansing they notice new discomfort. They couldn't notice it before because their circulation was so bad and the health of their nerve endings was so bad that they didn't really experience feeling in them. When they start getting life into the tissue, people start having new feelings, and they're a lot more sensitive to the condition of the body.

When I tell people about my seminars, I say, "Well, I'm going to have a seminar concerning gaining health and losing weight through internal cleansing." Then some will say, "Oh, yes. I need to lose some weight." Then I say, "Wait a minute. This one is on gaining health and losing weight."

They say, "Well, I'm pretty healthy; I have a few headaches now and then." Or, "Yes, I had a hysterectomy a few years ago." Or maybe, "Well, I've had my gallbladder removed, but I haven't had any trouble since." You see, ailments are so common today that people accept headaches, and one or two surgeries as being "pretty healthy."

In the medical profession, the most popular solutions so far have been drugs and surgery. In fact, some doctors seem to feel that they can remove all your problems in this way. For instance, consider little children who doctors are convinced should have their tonsils removed, even though tonsils are designed to handle toxins and fight infections.

Then they decide, "Well, it's about time the appendix came out." Yet the appendix is also designed to handle the overflow of toxins from the small intestine, and to fight infections.

Doctors can remove as much as one and a half lungs and you can still exist. They can remove your gallbladder. They can remove one kidney, or both kidneys. They can remove your spleen, three quarters of your stomach, your thyroid, and your colon. They can remove half of your heart. They can remove your eyes, your ears, arms, legs and all your sex organs, and the body will still exist. Hasn't science come a long way? They can cut all that out of you and you can still live. But actually, that is not living. That's just existing. If the body will still exist with all those parts missing, think what the body could do if it had all those parts functioning properly.

Removal of injured or infected body parts is not the type of internal cleansing I mean.

The body is designed with many precautionary methods of cleansing in case it gets poisoned. One problem we all face is that we have not grown up with the knowledge of how our body functions, nor what to do on a personal basis if it malfunctions. Also, we're in the jet age and people don't want to take time to cleanse. It has become so easy to just go to a doctor's office and say, "Well, I'm going on a trip next week. I have to be well. I have to be over this cold. Can't you just give me an antibiotic?" Or a person will develop gallstones and say, "Well, I don't have time to worry about correcting that. Just cut it out. I can recuperate and be on the road again." But more and more people are beginning to realize that is not the answer.

Some people have experienced unnecessary surgeries. For others the surgery they have had did more harm than good. Some people have taken prescription drugs that damaged them or turned them into drug addicts. Some of these people become bitter toward their doctors.

However, there is a fact we must remember: Everyone is responsible for his or her own health. If you're responsible for something, you must be educated about it in order to be able to make a reasonable decision. No one can force us to take drugs if we don't want them. No one can force us to have surgery we don't want. However, if we do not have knowledge about our bodies, we become easy prey for anyone who wants to involve us in unnecessary, unhealthful practices.

So if we are going to separate ourselves from the automatic drug and surgery syndrome, what is left as an alternative for health care? Internal Cleansing!!

I talk to a lot of women who have had female surgery and there is almost always a definite pattern. It starts with one ovary. The ovary had a cyst on it, so the doctor says, "We'll just take out that one ovary and that'll leave all the rest of your organs, so that won't be too bad."

Six months later, there's a cyst on the other ovary and the doctor says, "Boy, I was hoping this wouldn't happen, but it looks like we're going to have to take the other ovary. Well, as long as we're going in there to get that other ovary, we might as well take your uterus because you won't be able to have any more babies anyway and this will just save you another surgery later on."

In fact, they can convince you that they can save you money because they just take everything at one time. And if you do not understand the value of those organs, you are likely to agree to have them removed.

I knew of a similar experience with a customer in my restaurant. She told me, "I'm going in for surgery. I was going to go in for just some female surgery, but I've been having trouble with my gallbladder, so the doctor told me he'll just give me a good deal while he's in there." He was willing to take her female organs, her gallbladder, and her appendix all for the price of one operation. What a deal!

I said, "Well, you know, your recuperation's going to be quite a long time from that, counting your scar tissue and your mental scars." She said, "Oh, no. I know someone else who had this done and she said she never felt so good in all her life."

That's possible for a while. If you think about it, when a person's in terrible pain from a problem and then is drugged for a long period after surgery, you can actually feel better for a while.

But the problem is that once you've had the surgery, the results never end until you die. The years afterwards are never an improvement because the whole body works together. If you remove one thing, it definitely affects another. Just the scar tissue alone from the surgery can cause trouble.

When does it stop?

The only way to truly improve the condition of the body and nourish it properly is to cleanse and feed it according to its design. Ironically, at the same time you are cleansing and feeding your body properly, you will lose excess weight in the proper places.

I have had people pass 40 pounds of old feces from the colon. So if you want to lose weight, as well as cleanse, the removal of old feces would give you a pretty good start.

People say to me, "Well, I know that can't be my problem because I go to the bathroom every day, so I'm sure I don't have it."

I have news for you — everybody has it. When I weighed 105 pounds, I passed pounds of rubber-like feces. I passed a piece 3½-feet long when I went on a deep colon cleanse. And I had always gone to the bathroom every day and I had been cleansing for 10 years prior to doing that deep colon cleanse. (I will discuss this rubber-like feces and its formation in more detail later.)

There are visible signs to show us whether we have a problem internally or not. For instance, brown spots on the back of your hand, acne, eczema, or cellulite are all visible signs of putrefaction in the body. When you have putrefaction in the body, you have it in the colon.

You might wonder, "Well, wait a minute. If I have a bowel movement every day, why doesn't that stuff come out? How could it possibly stay in there?

One reason is that we have not been taught to wash the inside of the body enough. Many, many people seldom drink a glass of water. Most people who do drink water, drink some kind of city water that's putrefied. It's so bad, it's like taking a shower in soda pop. Also, most liquids that people drink are coffee, sodas or canned juices; things that do not wash the body. It has to be pure water.

Cigarettes, birth control pills, chemicals, wrong food combinations, food preservatives, internal menstrual pads, tight girdles, tight shorts, shallow breathing, polluted air, polluted water — all of these things contribute to a toxic body.

Now you don't have any control over some of these things. But, you do have control over nine out of ten of them. So if you keep those things that pollute your body out of your life, then you're only fighting one thing instead of ten.

We've been brainwashed, as far as losing weight is concerned, to either take appetite suppressants, count calories or have a high-protein, low-carbohydrate diet. All these methods are unnatural. They're unnatural for the body as far as nourishing it and as far as losing weight. In fact, many people today are suffering from health problems that are a result of some of the fad diets that they've tried.

If we continue to keep ourselves ignorant about how our bodies function, we will continue to be bilked out of our money with fad diets, fad drugs, and fad surgeries that have nothing to do with how the body works normally.

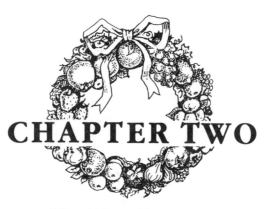

CHAPTER TWO

The Digestive Tract:
Our Basic Cleansing System

Since knowledge is necessary for you to be able to cleanse and eat properly, lets start with the basics.

On pages 10 and 11 is a picture of the digestive system, showing the digestive tract all the way from the mouth to the rectum.

Let's start at the mouth and go through the digestive process to see what is supposed to happen during the 18 to 24 hours that it normally takes to move food completely through your digestive system.

The digestive tract is open all the way through the body and it's approximately 30 feet long. Think of it: you're only about five or six feet tall, yet you have one part of your body that's 30 feeet long.

Now look at the chart. The digestive organs go down the center of your body and are designed to take in food, chew it, break it up, digest it, assimilate the nutrients and eliminate the indigestible parts, waste and residue. The digestive system then feeds these nutrients to the rest of the body. The whole body depends on what happens in the digestive tract.

There are muscles that are used all the way through the digestive tract. Some of those muscles propel food through it; some of them separate each step of the digestion, preventing food from backtracking. As the food goes further and further down the digestive tract, it gets smaller and smaller; at least, it's supposed to if everything's working right.

Food is no good to you unless it can be digested and assimilated. Undigested food poisons you and food that putrefies in your body is a major health problem throughout the world.

Each section of this digestive system has its own job and we have to make sure that it can take care of that job.

The Mouth

The first part is the mouth (Number 1 on the chart). I'm sure all of you have heard that you should chew your food well.

This is important with all foods, but especially carbohydrates. From the glands in the mouth saliva is secreted. When you have carbohydrates in your mouth, that saliva should contain an enzyme called ptyalin. That enzyme starts the digestion of carbohydrates in the mouth.

The Esophagus

The chart shows the esophagus, which is where the food goes directly from the mouth. In the esophagus (Number 2 on the chart) an action called the peristaltic action starts. Have you ever watched a worm wiggle like it's getting ready to do something, but it's not really doing anything? That's something like the peristaltic action. The movement goes on constantly, all through the digestive system, and that is the movement that moves the food through it.

The Cardiac Notch

Between the esophagus and the stomach, there's a muscle called the cardiac notch (Number 3 on chart).

DIGESTIVE SYSTEM

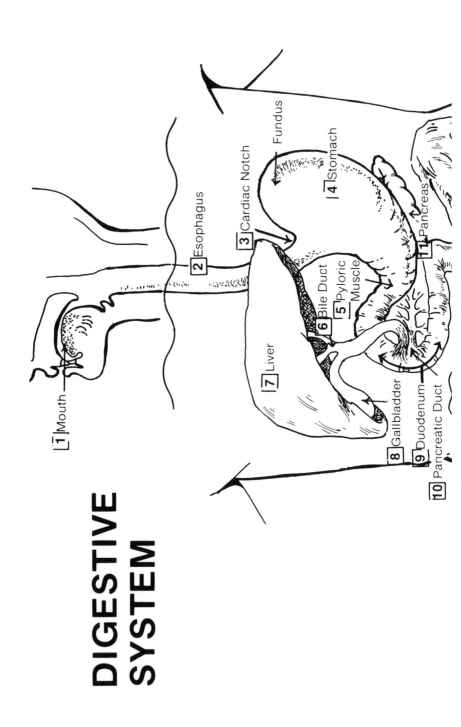

|1| Mouth
|2| Esophagus
|3| Cardiac Notch
Fundus
|4| Stomach
|5| Pyloric Muscle
|6| Bile Duct
|7| Liver
|8| Gallbladder
|9| Duodenum
|10| Pancreatic Duct
|11| Pancreas

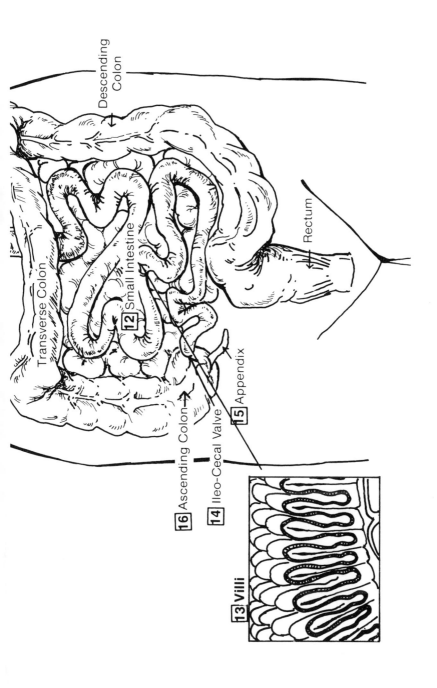

Descending Colon

Transverse Colon

Small Intestine **12**

Rectum

Ascending Colon **16**

Ileo-Cecal Valve **14**

Appendix **15**

Villi **13**

This notch closes after food enters the stomach. It's purpose is to prevent the food, once in the stomach mixing with the enzymes and digestive fluids, from returning to the esophagus.

Here's one of the first health problems that we find with digestion. Hydrochloric acid and pepsin are produced when you need to digest protein.

Let's say that you have some cheese (a protein) with salad (a proper combination) in your stomach mixed with the necessary acids and digestive enzymes. Then you add ice cream (*not* a proper combination) on top of it. That causes fermentation in the stomach, which in turn causes bloating and expansion of gas. It can become so bad, especially if you overeat, that it forces that cardiac notch to open, causing this total combination to back up into the esophagus. That results in an actual burning of the esophagus tissue because it has no protection from this combination.

The Stomach

The stomach (Number 4) is the only part of your body that has a protective lining to protect it from hydrochloric acid and pepsin. That's one reason we have muscles at both ends of the stomach. These muscles prevent food from backing up or leaving the stomach before its time. Since this very strong acid and pepsin combination is actually corrosive, it will burn any tissue outside the stomach.

You may be a person with an "acid stomach" and thinking you have too much acid, will take antacids to decrease the acid. That may not be the problem.

The problem may be that you do not have enough hydrochloric acid. In that case, every time you take an antacid, you're making the problem worse. What you may need to do, temporarily, is supplement with hydrochloric acid until the stomach is well enough and strong enough to produce it on its own. Then you can discontinue taking it.

By the way, if you do that, don't chew it in your mouth because it is an acid. Swallow it immediately so that it will get into the stomach where the protective lining is.

Sometimes people say to me after they've gone on a diet program, "Well, I can't eat as much as I used to be able to. I guess I've just shrunk my stomach." More likely the stomach has just gone back to its normal size. Many people do not realize that the stomach is like a balloon and it can expand and shrink.

Here is an example of that: I had a client who was very skinny in her legs and her buttocks, but she had a huge, huge belly. A doctor examined and checked her whole abdominal area. Now look at the chart and see where the stomach is supposed to be. Her stomach had stretched all over Numbers 9, 11, 12, and 16 on the chart. That's all over the pancreas, the duodenum, the small intestine and the ascending and transverse colon area.

If your stomach stretches that far, it only stretches because you have kept overeating and over-eating until you have permanently stretched it. That's what she had done over the years. Because it was so stretched, any time she ate, she never felt full. Think what a problem it's going to be for her to ever get her stomach back to its normal size.

This woman had a complete hysterectomy. A major cause of women having trouble with the uterus is the abnormal weight of the colon or of the stomach being stretched, which in turn puts such weight on the uterus that its own muscles can't hold it up anymore. It just collapses underneath the weight of the other organs.

You cannot stretch organs all over your body

wherever you want without affecting other organs. Now look at the top part of the stomach where the Number 3 is. It has the word "fundus" next to it. That part of the stomach toward the top is an open cavity. If you eat a meal and gas forms, the gas separates and goes to the top of your stomach area. When you burp, it comes from the top half of the stomach.

The Pyloric Muscle

The pyloric muscle (Number 5) is located in the bottom half of the stomach. This is the muscle that keeps food from leaving the stomach before it's fully digested.

If you didn't have that muscle and your stomach became full, the food could just keep passing on into the small intestine. But when you eat a meal and there's something to start digesting, that muscle contracts and holds itself closed until the food, or the parts of the food, have digested enough to enter the small intestine. The pyloric muscle will only open to release liquid, so the food must be in liquid form before passing into the small intestine.

Food is never assimilated through the stomach wall. Before I learned how the body works, I thought everything happened in the stomach. I thought the food digested there and it went into the system there and that's where you got all your nutrients. But that's not true.

However, there is one thing that does assimilate into the body through the wall of the stomach: alcohol. That's why a person can take a drink and in no time feel dizzy; the alcohol immediately goes through the wall of the stomach and into the bloodstream.

Digestion and Timing

Food digests in the stomach, depending upon what type of food it is, for two to 12 hours. Unfortunately, most people's eating schedule is something like this. For breakfast, they have coffee with cream (which requires 12 hours to digest) and sugar (a definite "no, no") or black coffee (another "no, no") and one slice of dry toast (which requires five hours). That might be at 7:00 in the morning. They go to work and they're on break at 10:00 — three hours later. They have some kind of breakfast roll (which will not digest no matter how long they wait) and another cup of coffee. They go to lunch and they have a sandwich (a combination which will putrefy) or a salad (probably with a dressing which will putrefy) at noon. Then they have a break in the middle of the afternoon at 2:00 or 3:00. They have another little snack then (which will mix in with the putrefied food still in the stomach). They go home and don't eat dinner until about 7;00 or 8:00 at night. Some don't eat dinner until 9:00 or 10:00 at night, just before they go to bed. This meal will also putrefy because there is not enough time between eating and going to bed.

In this schedule, not one meal all day long has been thoroughly digested. One reason is that before one meal could finish digesting, another meal landed on top of it.

For instance, suppose you have a slice of bread for breakfast. Even if it were the proper kind without sugar in it, it takes five hours to digest. But if you have it at 7:00 and you eat anything at all again before noon, even one piece of bread will not finish digesting. This sets up the putrefaction for the whole day. Therefore, all those meals which are constantly becoming toxic throw poisons into the system.

There are some people who have a blood sugar problem and temporarily have to adjust their eating so that they eat more often. But normally the body is not designed to eat long-digesting foods many times throughout the day.

If you ate just fruit many times a day, that would be a different story: the digestion time is only two hours, maybe three hours at the most. So you could eat every two or three hours and the food would be digested. But when you're eating cooked foods, and especially garbage foods that often take days to break down and pass through the body, it is impossible to digest them before adding another meal on top.

One thing that determines the time required for digestion is whether the food is cooked or raw. Raw food takes less time than cooked food because it still has digestive enzymes in it. Cooked foods take longer because as soon as you heat the food above approximately 105°F., it starts killing those enzymes. When they're all dead, your body has to produce all the necessary enzymes on its own to digest the food.

Digestion time depends both on what foods are eaten and what foods are eaten together. In the stomach wall, there are 35,000 glands that produce digestive aids. They produce gastric juice that is a mixture of mucus, enzymes, hydrochloric acid and a factor that enables the body to absorb vitamin B^{12} through the intestinal wall.

Pepsin and hydrochloric acid actually can disintegrate flesh and they do in order to break down meats. But it takes approximately 12 hours to do that and that is one reason why nations with a high consumption of meat are among the sickest people on earth. It just takes too much digestive time; it causes too much indigestion and the body is overtaxed.

Food and eating are supposed to be methods of helping the body cleanse internally. However, the modern day diet is so bad that now the whole body is called upon to eliminate the hazards created by our food and eating.

Drinking Liquids With Meals
Creates Three Major Problems

When I first tell people that, they say, "Wait a minute, Lee. I can't eat a meal without drinking a big glass of milk, or at least a big glass of juice, or a soda pop, or something like that."

They think they'll choke on the food. Indeed, they might, until they learn how to eat properly.

The first problem is that it prevents you from chewing the food as much as you should. That's why most people drink with their meals. They slap food in their mouths, chew it two or three times, and then want to swallow it right away. So they take a big swig of water, or milk, or something else, to get it down.

It is much better to eliminate the liquids and then chew the food until it is so liquid that it will swallow like water. That way you know you've chewed it enough and you have enough saliva in it. If it's a carbohydrate, you will probably have enough ptyalin in it; and then it's ready for the next step of digestion in the stomach.

The second problem is that liquids tend to dilute the digestive juices in the stomach. When those juices are diluted, they're not strong enough to break food down properly.

The third problem relates to the pyloric muscle (Number 5) that separates the steps of digestion between the stomach and small intestine. When foods have been broken down to pure liquids, that's a signal to the pyloric muscle to let some of the food out because it's completed that step of digestion. But when you drink liquids with the meal, it can trick that muscle and it can trick your stomach. The muscle thinks it's time to release some of the food. As a result, the liquid will leave the stomach. Because this liquid now has a high percentage of the digestive enzymes in with it, the enzymes leave the stomach with the liquid. What remains in the stomach is the solid, undigested food without the full complement of enzymes. This undigested, solid food can create problems.

To test these three problems, try eating without drinking liquids a few times and then try to drink with your meals again. You won't believe the difference in the way you will bloat when drinking with your meals, and the way you don't bloat when you don't drink liquids with them.

Liquids should never be taken closer than 15 minutes before eating, or for approximately two hours after eating. If your digestion time is slow and you're using my cleansing herbs, you might drink them 30 to 45 minutes before eating. That will give your slow digestion plenty of time to work before you consume any food. (Should you forget to take the herbs at least 15 minutes before eating, skip them for that meal only.)

Sometimes people ask if water is okay because I'm always preaching about making sure you get plenty of water. So they think, "Well, plain water must be okay with meals." However, water is a liquid, too. It has the same effect as far as diluting the enzymes and leaving the stomach before the food is properly digested.

Note: One way to tell if a meal was good or bad for you is whether or not it makes you thirsty. If it does, it was bad for you.

Let's review the digestive process so far. We chew our food well in the mouth. It goes down the esophagus into the stomach. Here the food is broken down to liquid form.

Remember, only the stomach has the protective mucous lining against hydrochloric acid. If the food is full of hydrochloric acid, it's only reasonable that something is going to have to happen to that food as it leaves the stomach to go into the duodenum.

And something does happen. A big change comes about here. Notice in your chart that the liver (Number 7), the gallbladder (Number 8) and the pancreatic duct (Number 10) join together right after the pyloric muscle.

If you will look at Number 9, which is the next part of the digestive tract right after the pyloric muscle, you will see that it is the part of the small intestine called the duodenum. Also leading into it is a duct (Number 6) which comes from the gallbladder and the liver. There's another duct coming from Number 11 (the pancreas) which also leads into it. There are many enzymes and digestive fluids that come into the duodenum (depending upon the food type) because they're all necessary for the next step of digestion.

The Liver

First of all, notice the liver (Number 7 on the chart). The liver weighs about four pounds. It comes from the right side, under the rib cage and across the middle of the abdomen.

The liver produces a liquid called bile and it sends the bile down to the gallbladder (Number 8) for storage. The liver aids digestion and the purpose of bile being stored is so that when fats leave the stomach, the gallbladder can squirt some of the bile into the digestive tract to emulsify, or break down, fats.

The liver also aids alkalinizaton of the intestine. Alkaline is the opposite of acid so any food coming out of the stomach which is acid will be neutralized in order to protect the rest of the digestive tract. What a wonderful design that the liver is located in just the right place to do this important job!

The liver also stores vitamins, and it stores digested carbohydrates. These must be digested and in the form of glucose sugar, which can be gradually released into the blood stream, to be used as energy. The liver also manufactures enzymes, particularly those that break down proteins.

In addition, the liver stores proteins, iron, copper and trace minerals. It stores vitamins A, D, E and the B vitamins. It stores blood coagulation factors, which are very, very important in case of injury and heavy bleeding. The liver not only stores blood coagulation factors, it also stores blood for emergencies. In addition, the liver "synthesizes" and stores amino acids. Synthesizes means that it puts the amino acids into a proper condition so that when they're needed, they can be used to build cells.

These amino acids are very important to our health. We have been taught that we must consume all essential amino acids at one time or none of them work. Therefore, we're told the best source of these acids is meat protein because it contains all the essential amino acids.

The liver keeps amino acids balanced in the body. This is how it works:

First of all, your body doesn't build cells from protein. In fact, it cannot build cells from protein. Protein must be converted to peptids and peptids must be converted to amino acids; then the body uses amino acids to build cells.

Many foods have amino acids in them, not just meat. Any source of amino acid can be used to build cells. These amino acids are taken into the body and they circulate in the blood and lymph system so that cells can be rebuilt as needed.

When there's an excess of any amino acid, the liver absorbs that excess and it stores it until needed. This stored supply in the liver contains all kinds of amino acids. When the amino acid level in the blood or the lymph drops due to the cells using it up, the liver will just send out the required ones and deposit them where they're needed.

So let's say that you ate a food that lacked two amino acids in order to provide a full balance. When you eat the food and it goes through the digestive tract, the body realizes that two amino acids are missing. The liver can release those two amino acids that are lacking to make up the balance. The next time you eat, maybe there are two different amino acids that are missing as the food goes through digestion. The body realizes which two are missing and again the liver will send out those two.

Some amino acids can be made by the body so nobody ever thinks of them as being a problem. However, there are some the body does not manufacture, so we must obtain them from our diet.

Natural foods, such as seeds, nuts, fruits and vegetables each contain some amino acids; but they don't each contain all of them. However, because of the body's built-in system of maintaining its balance of amino acids, it doesn't matter if you get them all in one food or not.

So when someone tells you, "Well, you're probably not getting enough protein," that might not be the problem. If you are eating dead, highly concentrated protein, the problem might be that you're not digesting that protein in order to get the amino acids. In such a case it's important to your health to change your diet to include foods that are easy to digest and to assimilate.

Foods that were originally designed for the body have protein in the form of lightweight protein molecules, or polypeptids. This form is easier for the body to digest and assimilate than the complex, hard-to-digest animal protein molecules.

I think it is very interesting also that "nature" reduces the amount of protein in human nursing milk from 2.38 percent (at birth) to 1.6 percent (within six months). At no other time of your life would you build more cells than during those six months and yet the protein decreases by 50 percent.

It is also very interesting that the decreased ratio of protein in nursing milk is almost identical to the protein ratio in green leafy vegetables. Think about that! Doesn't it seem reasonable in the design of things that the ratio of protein in natural foods should be a guide to us for the ratio of protein in our total diet?

A high protein diet, especially of dead animal food, is completely out of harmony with the original design of the body and its functioning.

Here's another point to consider: it is better to have a smaller amount of a nutrient and digest and assimilate it properly, than to eat a larger amount that putrefies in the digestive tract.

Dead foods, like meat, must putrefy to digest. In addition, most Americans are miscombining their foods and not getting the benefit of the amino acids that are in the protein because it never completely digests. As a result, you're better off to properly combine foods, and have a smaller amount of amino acids in a form that the body can use.

The bile that the liver produces also contains bile salts. These act like soap, or detergent, so that when fat comes from the stomach into the small intestine, it breaks down that fat.

An interesting point here is that the body never wastes anything. The design of it is remarkably efficient. After these bile salts are used to break down fats, they're reabsorbed and reused.

The bile also contains what is called bile pigment. Pigment has to do with color, and this is how it relates to bile: The bile disintegrates red blood cells and the residue of these used red blood cells is sloughed out of the body with waste. That puts color into your bowel movements. This color can help you determine your general state of health and whether the liver and bile are functioning properly. If your bowel movements are white, the bile or liver is not functioning properly.

The liver also works with vitamin C to control alcohol in the body.

On occasion I've had someone say to me, "Lee, I went to the doctor. He says I have cirrhosis of the liver and I have never drunk alcohol in my whole life."

How in the world can this happen?

If you eat carbohydrates and they ferment in your stomach, they turn into alcohol. To the body that's the same as if you had a stiff drink. The body doesn't say, "Oh, well, this alcohol came from indigestion. It's okay." Many people who believe it is a sin to drink alcohol gorge themselves on poisonous carbohydrates such as cakes, pies, cookies and candies. Or they eat fruits at the wrong time, and with the wrong food combinations. All of these turn into alcohol. Your body doesn't care if it came from a liquor bottle or the cake plate. If it's alcohol, it's alcohol; the damage is the same.

Another thing the liver does is to detoxify drugs, poisons and chemicals. If you slice the liver across the grain, you see that it has minute holes in it. The whole liver is like a sieve. It's weblike and it sieves toxins that go through it. It can completely filter those out if it is working properly.

But what amazes me about the liver is that it not only cleans, but it's a warehouse, too. Then, after it cleans and stores all these important ingredients in digestion, it feeds the body whenever the body needs what it's storing. The liver is truly a marvelous organ.

The Gallbladder

Next on the chart is Number 8, the gallbladder. It hangs right underneath the liver. There is a duct that joins them together. That's how the liver sends bile to the gallbladder. That duct (Number 6) also proceeds to the duodenum in order for the bile to be added to any fat foods that are coming from the stomach, as well as to neutralize the acid from the stomach.

The gallbladder is only about three inches long, yet it modifies the bile tenfold. In other words, it condenses the bile so that it becomes ten times stronger than when it comes out of the liver. Then, when food comes from the stomach that needs to have bile added, the gallbladder puts bile into the duodenum — at just the appropriate time.

Many people have gallstones, but don't know it until these gallstones start moving. Gallstones are calcified, sharp and hard. If an x-ray should determine you have stones, and you're in pain, do you know what most doctors will recommend? That you have that little organ removed.

The *Better Homes & Garden Family Medical Guide,* prepared by "a corps of medical men which includes several of America's most distinguished medical authorities and specialists," says on page 479 under the *Gallbladder* heading:

"The gallbladder is a sac-like structure which stores and concentrates the bile which is constantly being secreted by the liver. The gallbladder is not essential to health."

Hogwash!

Where will you store bile if you don't have a gallbladder? If fatty foods and acid foods leave the stomach and they need that strong bile, will you have the proper reaction there without a gallbladder? No.

And what is more ridiculous is that even without a gallbladder, you don't solve the gallstone problem, because you can still develop gallstones without a gallbladder.

In my cassette album, *Cleansing vs. Surgery*, I teach a special gallbladder cleanse which I have used myself. Thousands of other people have also used it and have passed thousands of gallstones without pain. In fact, I have passed more than 500 of them and, until I did that cleanse, I didn't even know I had them. Some people scheduled for gallbladder surgery decide at the last minute, "Well, maybe I'll take a chance; I'll do this cleanse. If it works, fine. If not, I'll go ahead and have the surgery."

Can you imagine what a phenomenal thing it is for a person to be scheduled for surgery, do the gallbladder cleanse, which is completely painless, and never have to have the surgery? You can always have the gallbladder removed, but you can't ever get it back once it's out.

The expense of the gallbladder cleanse is approximately $15; it takes 3 days at the most, and there's no pain when the stones come out. Compare that to a $9,000 surgery, weeks of recuperation, scar tissue for the rest of your life and living without a gallbladder.

Even people who have had their gallbladders removed use the gallbladder cleanse and still pass as many as 50 to 100 gallstones. What good did it do them to have the gallbladder removed? When the gallbladder is removed, the space leaves a little pocket, and the same health problem continues to exist. So the stones keep forming. These stones are usually of hardened fat, bile and crystals which do not break down because of a malfunction of the digestive system. But bile comes from the liver and you have to stop production of bile if you don't want gallstones to form. So, following the currently popular medical reasoning, you would have to take the liver out too.

While in the gallbladder the stones are calcified, but once they leave the gallbladder, they start to melt down. That's how I lost my first 300 stones. I dug them out of the toilet, but I didn't know they would melt. I had them in a jar and the next day when I was going to show them to some people, they were all fused into one big glob of fat-like bile in the jar. So if you want to save your gallstones after you pass them, you have to keep them in the freezer. And believe me, you will enjoy showing them to other people.

The Pancreas

Number 11 on the chart is the pancreas. This gland is about six inches long. The pancreas aids digestion as well as functioning as an endocrine gland. (An endocrine gland shoots fluid directly into the blood stream.)

Many people are familiar with the pancreas because of the symptom diabetes. Now look on the chart; the pancreas extends from the left side of the body to the right immediately under the stomach. It's a long, skinny organ. Down the middle of the pancreas there is a dark line, which is a duct called the **pancreatic duct** (Number 10). In that duct, enzymes are secreted as well as a watery, mucousy substance. These different enzymes (which go directly into the digestive tract) further break up fats, proteins and carbohydrates so that the body can digest them.

That duct comes out at the same point where the gallbladder and the liver duct join the duodenum. All of these digestive organs come together right there at the same point where they are needed for the next step of digestion after the food leaves the stomach.

The pancreas also produces insulin. However, the insulin does not go directly into the digestive system. The pancreas squirts insulin directly into the bloodstream in order to regulate the use of the sugar already in the blood.

In addition, the pancreas produces bicarbonate neuters. Many people take bicarbonate of soda to neutralize acids. The neuters in the pancreas use the same principle, so you should never need to add them to your digestive system.

An interesting point here is that if a person has trouble with either the liver, gallbladder or pancreas, one can almost be sure to have trouble with the others. This is because they accent each other and rely on each other. That's one of the main problems with having the gallbladder removed. If the gallbladder is removed, eventually you're going to have liver and pancreas problems. People who have had their gallbladder removed should make a special effort to keep their liver and pancreas working properly, since those two organs have to take some of the load that the gallbladder carried.

For example, suppose you broke a leg and had to walk with crutches. You could still walk, but the leg that you're using all the time will tire and wear out faster until the other one heals. That's how it works with the pancreas, gallbladder and liver combination.

The main problem is that once you've had an organ removed, there's no going back. I encourage anyone with any problem in the digestive system to please try cleansing first.

I want to give you an example of how you can rejuvenate the body even if it's deteriorated to the point where an organ is hardly functioning.

A woman came to me about three years ago. She was eating only 350 calories daily and had been on that diet for six months. She was overweight — the original reason for that ridiculous program — but even at 350 calories a day, she actually gained weight. She was a nervous wreck; she couldn't digest her food, and her thighs were bulging.

This was her diet: she was eating one piece of broiled meat and one piece of fruit every day. Every time she ate, she would bloat with gas so badly that she had to unzip her pants and open them to relieve the pressure.

Through education about her body, she started concentrating on rehabilitating her digestive organs. It took her 3½ months to be able to digest any food at all, even using Proper Food Combining. She gradually increased her food intake to three full meals per day. It was at that point that her weight loss started. Her body eventually normalized. This case involved a young woman, so it did not take a long time to rejuvenate her body, but the older we are and the longer we've had the problem, the longer it takes to correct it.

The exciting thing is this: each day you're on a cleansing program and using Proper Food Combining, the body does experience improvement. What more can we want out of life? Think how encouraging it is mentally and spiritually to think each day that you are getting better instead of worse.

One of the worst things for your health is to know that every day you're getting worse. You can wake up thinking, "Well, today I'm just going to be worse. What's the sense of trying?" It's important not to get discouraged. Be patient!

One time I lived on just juices for almost a year. *Don't try it.* You can get mighty hungry to chew something when all you've had is juices for a whole year. But every day I felt better and I lost more weight, especially cellulite weight. Those results encouraged me to stay on that program. As you start feeling better and as these toxins start leaving, realize it is going to take a while to gain your health back and lose the weight. But it will happen!

Another thing I want you to keep in mind — sometimes surgery and drugs can seem like they are easier and faster. You think you'll correct the problem, but you have no idea what having one surgery can create in terms of other problems that can originate in the body. The recuperation time is the rest of your life. So, why not just make up your mind to cleanse for a few years, a few months even, and perhaps save yourself the pain and expense of drugs and surgery?

The Duodenum

The next part we're going to discuss is the duodenum. That's Number 9 on your chart. The duodenum is approximately eight to 10 inches long. Notice on the chart (pages 10 and 11) how it starts descending; it curves to the side, continues down and becomes Number 12, the small intestine.

Keep in mind that if the food arriving at the duodenum, is highly acid, it becomes alkaline at this point due to the work of the pancreas, the liver and the gallbladder. If they work properly, there's no problem.

The Small Intestine

Next the food moves on to the small intestine. This is Number 12 on the illustration. This part of the 30-foot-long tube is approximately 20 feet long. It has a mucous lining and inside there are about 5 million finger-like villi.

On page 30, the illustration shows the villi. They face in toward the center of the intestine and increase the surface of the intestinal wall for absorption. In fact, the internal surface area of the small intestines is more than five times that of the body's entire skin surface.

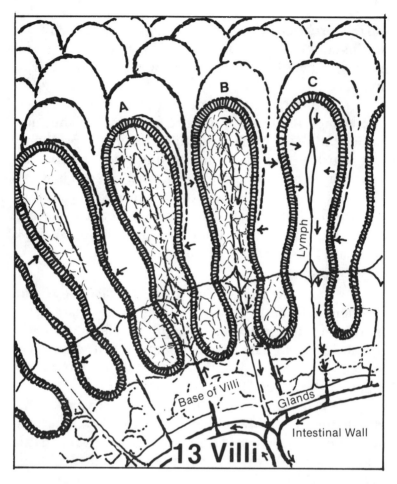

Base of Villi

Glands

Lymph

Intestinal Wall

13 Villi

Notice on the illustration of the villi that there are three different phases of the absorption. This illustration shows the three different steps that happen in this area. The left one (A) shows arrows going into it; the middle one (B) shows arrows coming out, and the one on the right (C) shows them coming in from the side. Notice the squares at the base of the villi. The arrows going into the villi denote the blood supply going in to feed the villi, because blood takes the nutrients (or toxins) to the tissue. The one coming out is your blood supply picking up nutrients (or toxins) from the villi. You see how the blood just keeps rotating in these all the time — pick up, delivery, pick up, delivery. The arrows going sideways indicate absorption into the villi through the wall.

Notice the squares at the base of the villi. This is where it is attached to the wall of the intestine. At the base of the villi are glands that secrete alkaline juices, enzymes and mucus.

The villi are always moving. They sway back and forth, like wheat blowing in the wind. This motion is the reason for something we hear everyday. Have you ever heard anyone with rumbling noise in their abdomen? They say, "Oh, my stomach is growling." That is not the stomach. It's the small intestine where the villi are; it's the villi moving that causes that growling noise. If you hear something from the stomach, it's a burp.

On pages 10 and 11, notice that the intestine winds back and forth, up and down and all around in layers.

I want to explain this to you. The back of this 20-foot-long tube is attached to what is called the mesentery wall. To visualize that, spread your hand wide open and look directly at the palm of your hand. That's what the mesentery wall is like; it's what holds the small intestine in place. The wall is flat and it's attached to the back of the abdomen area. It is loaded with blood and lymph capillaries, which carry nutrients, or poisons, back from the wall of the small intestine into the rest of the body. This wall is loose — it's very flexible and it permits freedom of movement by the slippery intestine.

Most nutrients are absorbed into the body through lymph and blood capillaries in the wall or villi of the small intestine. These feeder lymph and blood capillaries that start from the wall of the intestine lead to larger capillaries. Food which is in the stomach isn't even close to being ready for assimilation. It has to pass the gallbladder, the liver and the pancreas, and then it goes down into the small intestine where it is processed in the final step of digestion.

By the time the small intestine finishes its job, the food should be so broken down and so minute that it will seep through the villi wall. After the nutrients go into the villi, they eventually seep back to larger and larger capillaries and veins and eventually reach the liver. Then in the liver they are reduced down even further and the digested food is then delivered from the liver to other parts of the body, whenever it's needed.

The Ileo-Cecal Valve

Between the small intestine and the large colon is a valve called the ileo-cecal valve (Number 14). It's located where the feces comes from the small intestine into the colon. The purpose of this valve is to keep the food from seeping back into the small intestine after it's in the colon.

The Appendix

Find the place on the chart where the small intestine and the large colon come together.

At the bottom of the colon is a small organ hanging down that's about three inches long. That's the appendix (Number 15).

People with their appendix have an advantage over those who don't. Here's why: Any time a toxin leaves the small intestine to move into the colon, the appendix squirts out a germicidal mucus designed to destroy poisons or toxins.

Due to the diets of most people today, and as sick as we are, there are toxins that enter the colon every day. I've seen pictures of appendices that were so inflamed that they actually became as large in circumference as the colon. Continual putrefaction leaving the small intestine causes the appendix to overwork in its efforts to keep the large colon poison free. Also, worms and toxins tend to gather and lay in the natural pocket at the bottom of the colon adjoining the appendix. Removal of the appendix is not in harmony with the body's design. Cleansing is!

Ascending, Transverse, and Descending Colon

The next organ is the colon. That is Number 16 on the digestive tract chart.

The colon, on the left side of the chart, which is the right side of your body, is the ascending colon, and it goes up to the rib cage. It then crosses over to the left side of your body and that part is called the transverse colon. Then it comes down the left side of your body and that section is called the descending colon.

Years ago when I had terrible health problems, x-rays showed that my ascending colon only rose about a quarter of the way up where it should have been, and that the transcending and descending sections were prolapsed and laying in the left hip pocket. My whole colon was so infected and toxic it was poisoning me to death. With deep muscle massage, Proper Food Combining and other internal cleansing, my colon is now normal. How much better than removing the colon and wearing a colostomy bag!!

The colon is close to five or six feet in length and is normally about 2½ inches in diameter. However, most people's colon is not normal. The chart shows the normal size and the normal way that it hangs. Some people's colons are so stretched and out of place that they're almost twice as long as normal. And some people's are so swollen and so loaded with old feces that sections are twice as large in diameter as they should be. On the other hand, some of them haven't worked for so long that they're really skinny in areas and the feces can barely move through them.

As the chart shows, the outside of the colon looks like it has bulges on it. Those are muscles. These muscles are supposed to constantly contract so that they continually move feces through the colon.

If there were no strong muscles there to continually do that, the feces would lay there until another meal arrived behind it to shove it out. That is exactly what's happening with many people.

Constipation and its Remedies

Many people will not admit they are constipated. It is not a subject generally discussed in public.

Nonetheless, there are 45,000 laxatives on the market. *Somebody* must be constipated.

I did a survey of my female clients to which 75 percent responded that they had a bowel movement only once every two weeks. They all reported how rotten they felt: they were always bloated; they couldn't lose weight; their pants didn't fit. They'd have to unzip their pants after every meal. One thing they had in common was that they had all talked to their doctors about it and all of their doctors said, "Don't worry about it; you've been that way all your life. It's just normal for you."

In two weeks you eat about 42 meals. If you only have one bowel movement where are the other 41 meals? Not only is it abnormal to have only one bowel movement every two weeks, it's also abnormal to have to take laxatives. Statistics show that *at least* 25 percent of all Americans take a laxative two to three times a week.

Once in a while when someone changes their eating habits they become constipated. Actually they had been constipated all along, they just didn't know it.

These people's colon muscles have not really worked for a long time. Because the colon muscles were unaccustomed to working it took a large volume of feces to keep shoving out the previous feces. Thus, if they reduce their volume of food, or change to other food types, the volume has to accumulate to reach the level to which the colon is accustomed.

The answer to this problem is — stick with it. Stick with the cleansing and the food combining because eventually these old pockets will move out. By the discontinuance of toxins piling up, the muscles actually will start functioning again in most cases. The temporary use of an herbal laxative has helped most problem cases make the transition.

Another point that is important to remember is how long it takes food to go through your digestive tract. One way to find out how your body digests is to be able to identify that food.

Normally it takes 18 to 24 hours for food to be completely assimilated and removed. If you eat foods that you can identify in the stool, it won't be any problem for you to check the timing. For instance, beets are a bright purple color, so eat some beets and wait and see how long it is before these beets come out in your bowel movement. That way, you'll know how long your food is taking to digest. Corn is another indicator because its residue is indigestible. Learn how to identify your waste so you can keep a check on the health of your digestive tract.

Once the body begins to cleanse, it is helpful to be able to identify the old feces. I recently had a man tell me, "Lee, there's no problem with that. As long as I have a nose, I'll be able to identify the old feces."

We have had people tell us they pass bowel movements that are 20 years old and you may wonder how we know that.

Remember when the low carbohydrate diet first

became popular? That was about 20 to 25 years ago. One of the foods that people on that program stopped eating was corn because it was high in carbohydrates. I have had many people use our cleanse and say, "You won't believe this. I had a bowel movement yesterday with corn in it and I haven't eaten corn for 20 years."

They're usually amazed when I can describe exactly what that old corn feces looked like. It's always surrounded by a coating of thick, dark, yellow-brown mucus slime and it has a tail on it, like some kind of fish. You see, that toxin starts building around the corn kernels and over the years it builds more and more.

If the corn is still there, how do we know the rest of the meal isn't? The fact is that some of it is still there. It just can't be identified as easily as corn. When you pass old feces, the gas, the odor and the fumes are all so toxic that you can hardly stand it.

You could take the attitude, "I'm not doing this cleansing stuff. Are you kidding? I'm not going around passing this stinking gas."

But what if it stays in there?

To start with, for a few years, it will just lay there and fester. As it seeps back into the digestive tract and the eliminative organs, and they can't handle it, you will find more of your organs will not function properly. When it gets back to the cell level throughout the whole body, you'll be able to see it one way or another.

Diverticulitis

In some cases, the colon will develop a pocket bulging in the colon wall. This is known as diverticulitis. The longer the pocket exists, the less the muscle structure in the wall can work. The less it works, the larger the pocket becomes.

In fact, I've seen x-rays of pockets that have been 10 to 12 inches in circumference, instead of the normal

2½ inches. Those pockets are full of old feces and toxins of all sorts, and are highly dangerous to your health.

If one of these diverticulitis bulges should burst, the poisons could flood the body so fast that it could be fatal.

Most people do not realize the extent of danger of diverticulitis. I've had people come to me and once the pain is gone, they're back to their old eating habits.

It is important to note that the colon does not have a lot of nerves in it. Sometimes it is difficult to know what's happening in the colon. Because of a lack of nerve endings, you don't feel pain as easily as you would in other parts of the body. So if you do have pain there, you know you really do have a problem. On the other hand, the lack of pain does not necessarily mean the problem has been corrected. If something is numb or deadened, it has no pain.

The lining of the colon has lymph and blood capillaries which lead to different parts of your body. For instance, there are capillaries leading back to your eyes. If your colon is highly impacted or infected in that area, eventually your eyesight will be affected by it. On the other hand, cleanse the colon thoroughly in that area and many people experience an improvement in their vision.

A final residue of nutrients is the only thing that should pass through the wall of the colon. However, when the colon lining is clogged with 20- to 30-year-old feces, what nourishment could go through the lining?

Instead of nourishment, toxins seep into the colon-lining capillaries and eventually seep back to various parts of the body. If these toxic parts of the colon are discovered and are cleaned, you will eventually see an improvement in the part of the body affected by the colon.

There are two reasons why we don't notice these problems until they're critical:

Firstly, this is a gradual deterioration, so you don't feel it because it doesn't just build overnight. It's so gradual that we just adapt to it.

Secondly, we are so ignorant of our bodies that we don't even suspect anything like this could be developing.

For example, consider the mucous lining of the colon.

Most people don't even know it exists, let alone that they are breeding a whole field of toxic gases, mucus, poisons and feces in that mucous lining. This mucous lining becomes a fertile ground for unhealthy bacterial life forms, which then begin multiplying. As time passes, this lining gets thicker and thicker like adding cornstarch to a thickened sauce, and it takes on the consistency of rubber.

As I mentioned previously, I passed bits and pieces of this rubber-like mucus while on a colon cleanse. I also passed a piece 3½ foot long that looked just like a colon. This rubber-like mucus does not break apart and cannot be cut. You can actually hold it up in the air and it will react like a tough rubber band.

Friendly bacteria must be constantly present in the digestive tract to destroy unfriendly bacteria. Friendly bacteria (most commonly known today as acidophilus) get conquered by the excess of "un-friendly" bacteria in this mucus. When that happens you have lost a major natural cleansing process.

After food has finished processing in the colon, there are by-products left. One is called scatol. This is very foul-smelling. There's also hydrogen sulfide, fatty acids, methane gas, and carbon dioxide. In fact, more than 36 highly toxic poisons have been found to exist in the colon. These by-products are a result of the extensive deterioration of Man's health and eating habits.

The Lymph — An Associate Cleansing System

Since the lymph is such an important part of our cleansing, I want to discuss it in more detail. The body contains three quarts of blood. It also contains 12 quarts of lymph — or four times as much lymph as blood. The lymph system and all its capillaries (see the illustration on page 41) is completely separate from the blood system and its capillaries.

Blood moves quickly through capillaries, but the lymph moves slowly through capillaries. A major function of the blood is to take nutrients to the cells. A major function of the lymph is to pick up toxins and waste to take them away from the cell. It is a normal body function for waste and residue to be continually sloughed off at the cellular level. Hence, by way of the lymph system, the body is, or is supposed to be, cleansing constantly.

Look back at the diagram of the villi on page 30 and you'll notice the one on the right (C) shows a feeder in the middle. These feeders are part of the lymph. Digested fat is assimilated into the body through these feeders. Every villi has a lymph feeder down the middle of it which feeds back to larger lymph capillaries.

Fatty foods, when digested, follow a path back through the lymph system. It takes them from the lymph feeder to the lymph system, which goes back through the mesentery wall, and eventually leads to a duct called the thoracic duct. This is a main lymph channel that goes up the front of the spinal column. This channel collects lymph from various parts of the body, and then empties the lymph into the vena cava, which is in the neck area. From the vena cava, it enters the bloodstream, and nutrients go to the liver for final processing. Digested carbohydrates and proteins travel through the blood capillaries to the portal vein to the liver. Then all digested food substances can be delivered to cells of the body as needed.

Regardless of whether it is fat, protein or carbohydrates, food must be very minute to pass through the intestinal wall.

If your body does not digest your meals and you have toxins laying in the small intestine or the colon, these toxins can travel back through the blood or lymph system. It doesn't have to be just nutrients; poisons can also be assimilated in those villi in the small intestine.

The tonsils and the appendix are lymph organs, and designed to help cleanse internally.

These are the very organs that the medical association has said we no longer need. As a result, doctors have removed them from people's bodies as though they had no importance.

Here's what *The Better Homes And Gardens Family Medical Guide*, (Revised Edition, 1980) says about the appendix on page 489, under *Appendicitis*. "The appendix is a vestigial organ." (Vestigial means it was useful at one time, but it no longer is.) Continuing to quote, "It is a vestigial organ of no use to human beings. It is only important when it becomes inflamed and infected. Immediate surgery is then necessary to remove the appendix."

The New Illustrated Family Medical and Health Guide, by the Editors of Consumer Guide (1984) states on page 233, under the heading *Appendicitis,* "Although it may have had a function at some point in human development, the appendix serves no purpose now."

HOGWASH!!

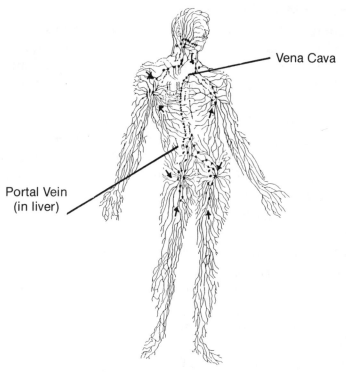

Vena Cava

Portal Vein
(in liver)

LYMPH SYSTEM

Doctors apparently feel the same way about the tonsils, which is why they have continued to remove them from millions of people over the years.

However, a long-range survey shows that it is very hard to maintain health when you have had your tonsils and your appendix removed. Removal of infected overburdened lymph organs is not internal cleansing according to the body's design. Feeding, washing and rejuvenating these organs is.

The lymph plays an important part in internal cleansing. The lymph only moves in one direction. From the feet it moves up to the chest area. In the groin and in the abdomen area, on the side of the breasts and under the armpits, and in the neck, there are hundreds of lymph nodes. The nodes are small and round, and are designed to disintegrate any toxins in the lymph system. The lymph fluid passes through these nodes, the nodes destroy any toxins in the lymph and as the lymph fluid leaves the nodes, it should be clean and contain some self-protecting white blood cells.

The problem is that the body becomes over-toxic. As a result the nodes are overworked and they can't handle the job. Thus, when the lymph fluid becomes overloaded and cannot remove the toxins from around the cells, everything becomes overloaded. The eliminative organs, such as the kidneys, the liver, the skin, and the bowel, can't function properly if the lymph is overloaded. When all of these organs don't function properly, toxins back up in them, which backs up the poison all the way to the cell level throughout the body.

The problem is expanded if you have had organs removed.

When toxin is backed up at the cell level, it stops what's called the sodium-potassium pump. Every single cell must have that pump activity in order for it to live: it is impossible to have life in a cell without the sodium-potassium pump working.

Inside each cell, there should be an amount of potassium, iron, calcium, glucose, and other nutrients. Outside each cell, around it, there should be an amount of sodium. This combination sets up a pump action which creates an electrical flow.

But when there's an overflow of toxins dumped at the cell level by circulating blood, excess sodium invades the cells. The pump activity is stopped and circulation becomes very poor. The toxins flood the tissue because the lymph can't pick up as fast as the blood is dumping. Excess water and toxins eventually burst or expand those cells and when there are thousands of them, you see it as cellulite and/or obesity. (For further explanation, see *The Golden Seven Plus One*, by C. Samuel West.)

One of the main reasons obesity settles in the legs, thighs and buttocks is because lymph moves uphill in the legs. Naturally, anything going up requires more effort than something coming down. So when the lymph tries to come up from the legs and the circulation is already poor, it can't do it. The result is that toxins settle in the poor circulation areas.

The Visible Evidence of Toxins

Most people are like I am: until the toxins in my body became cellulite and obesity, I wasn't all that worried about them. Most excess weight is poison weight. Since this is the case, it would only make sense, that if we reverse that and eliminate the poisons, the excess weight will be gone.

Think for a minute. Do you have any weight on your body that you want to eliminate? If so, how does it look naked? There's where we really see the proof, isn't it? Even though most people aren't going to see you naked, the point is you will. And you're the one who will be analyzing your progress and you must *know* your body in order to do that.

So is your fat puckered? Does it hang? Is it lumpy? How does it look with your clothes on? Is it still puckered, lumpy and does it still hang? Haven't we all seen someone wearing a pair of slacks and we could actually see the rippled, ugly fat right through it? That's a very visible sign of toxic weight. When the poisons go, the puckered, lumpy, rippled fat goes.

The amazing part is, you don't really *see* the root cause of your toxic weight because you've had it inside the body long before you ever saw it on the outside.

I've had clients come to me who've been eating only 500 calories a day. They would lose weight because they were actually starving their bodies to death, but they still had bulging problem areas.

That's when they'd say to me, "Lee, my arms get thin, I lose my breast tissue, my stomach goes flat, but I still have big thighs." You see, losing healthy tissue through starving the body is not the same as cleansing. When you lose weight through cleansing, you only lose the bad stuff and you keep the good.

With a little help from herbs, the body can start to eliminate the root cause of your visible toxic weight and you will not only be thinner and look better, but you will feel better, act better and be better.

Obesity is so serious to us that many people would rather have cancer than be fat.

For example, haven't we all heard people say, (and I said it to myself years ago), "Well, I would quit smoking, but I'm afraid I'll gain weight." Many people recognize the danger of smoking and the health problems associated with it, and yet would rather take a chance with their health than gain weight.

Let's analyze that.

Think of all the people you know who smoke: Are they all nice and thin with no toxic fat? The obvious answer is "no." Apparently continuing to smoke is not the way to be thin and healthy. As a matter of fact, smoking is one of the major causes of cellulite because of the huge amount of toxic buildup that it causes in the body.

Another example involves diet drinks. The ingredients in diet drinks can actually cause your kidneys and bladder to malfunction. Yet people will drink them daily to keep their weight down. If damage is done to the kidneys, a person can actually gain weight consuming diet drinks.

So let's think about that. Do all people who drink diet sodas get rid of their weight problem? Or are they still fighting the battle of the bulge?

Once again, the answer is obvious — most people we know who are drinking diet sodas to control their weight still have a weight problem.

Sometimes women say to me, "Well, you know I never had cellulite until I had my last baby." It wasn't their eating habits or putrefaction; it was the child. Or they say, "Yes, I have big thighs, Lee, but that's just like my mother. I have four sisters and we all have these big cellulite bags." That makes it her mother's and her sister's fault. It wasn't anything she ate.

Let's be honest about it, and let's face it: poisons in our body are the cause of this problem.

It is true that we can inherit some toxins from birth. But as we grow older, most of us tend to continue eating and living with habits like our parents' and that's why the same problem exists. If we change our eating and living habits, we find that it is not an inherited problem and it will go away.

The fact that all women in the same family have big thighs and obese legs merely means they *all* need internal cleansing.

I work with a lot of women's massage salons which specialize in getting circulation into the problem areas. Some of them say when they first start working on some women, the pockets in the cellulite areas are so deep that they can actually stick their fingers all the way in. Those women are extremely toxic. Internal cleansing is an urgent matter for them and I don't mean just for a month and then back to the old habits; I mean for the rest of their lives.

The usual visible evidence of obesity, or toxic weight, usually includes a large, protruding abdomen, bags (often called saddlebags) on the thighs, especially on women, or swollen ankles. The major places where problem weight forms are the areas of the body where there is poor circulation.

In addition to obesity many of us, at one time or another, have had allergies, hay fever, bad tonsils, appendicitis, gout, diabetes, gallstones, hepatitis, varicose veins, arthritis, menstrual problems, female problems, cysts, acid stomach, age spots on the hands, bad breath, a cold, constipation, water retention, eczema, exhaustion, fever, gas, hemorrhoids, high blood pressure, hypoglycemia, itch, kidney stones, acne and so on.

The truth is that all the *illnesses* I have just listed are symptoms of the same problem. They are all caused by putrefaction and constipation throughout the body. They are all basically caused by toxic waste in the body, which causes all organs and body functions to become so congested with toxic mucus that they will not function properly.

Remember, the whole body works together. If one organ is malfunctioning, it will cause a load on other organs and eventually they will malfunction. They, in turn, will cause a load on other organs and they will malfunction. In time, this putrefaction throughout the body becomes so extensive that your eliminative organs cannot handle it. So it settles in poor circulation areas of the body and when we see it visibly, we call it cellulite and obesity, or some illness.

A congested body, a putrid body, is the root cause of your health problems. Knowledge of how the body functions, what cleansing it needs, and how to feed it properly is a *must*!!

The Invisible Toxic Storehouses

The unseen toxic pounds on the body are usually located in three areas.

First, the colon. As noted above, I have known cases in which people's colons contained up to 40 pounds of old feces. There is no way in the world that a body could not be full of poisons with a colon that congested.

The second area is the kidneys. The kidneys can hold pounds of liquids. In fact, many people find that once they get into a serious body cleansing program they discover that their kidneys have been polluted with pounds of old toxic waste. Some people pass urine which is so full of mucus, it is "thick."

The kidneys are designed to separate toxins from the body's fluids, and eject the toxins from the body. The kidneys, therefore, are part of the original internal cleansing program.

While the kidneys can hold pounds of liquids and toxins, that was not their original purpose. In spite of these toxins, they still can function somewhat.

One thing we've noticed is that we have had many people who started to lose weight on daily mild cleansing and all of a sudden their weight loss stops. This usually happens after they have lost approximately 10 pounds and/or in approximately 30 days. If they go on the kidney cleanse, a deeper special cleanse, they not only lose up to 15 pounds in three days, but they continue to lose weight after going off the cleanse. (Refer to my *Cleansing vs. Surgery* cassette tape.)

I have had many people do my kidney cleanse and while straining their urine during the cleanse they discover that they passed many kidney stones. These are people who did not even know they had kidney stones. They had no idea that their kidneys were not functioning properly. Some had backaches for years and did not realize that the backache was coming from a kidney that was in pain.

The third main toxic storehouse is the tissue throughout the body at the cellular level.

A body can hold up to 80 pounds of toxic water. When excess blood proteins escape into the tissues, excess water follows them and floods each cell. (An example is water retention after eating salty foods.) Since the lymph moves slowly it cannot pick up the excess and this fluid lays in the cells until you make an extra effort to remove it.

Sometimes when people go on a cleanse, their tissue is so loaded with toxins and water that they will lose as much as 25 pounds in a week. They live "on the toilet." Many people say, "Well, that's just water loss." No, it is not just water loss. It is water and *poison loss*. When you get rid of that, the body immediately starts functioning better.

This weight loss has nothing to do with cutting your calories by 3,500 calories in order to burn off a pound of weight. It has to do with cleansing the body at the cellular level to help your whole system function better.

To give you an example, I had a client who had thighs that were loaded with cellulite. I saw her on a Friday, and her slacks fit so tightly the seams were pulling. She was 100 pounds overweight.

She went on my herbal cleanse, lots of steam-distilled water, and fruits and vegetables. She came back five days later wearing the same pair of slacks, which hung on her like a gunny sack.

She had dropped 25 pounds during these five days and she told me that her urine color was extremely dark for the first two days. It had such a terrible, smelly odor she left the bathroom window open. But by the fifth day, she had seen a tremendous difference in the color of the urine and in the odor of it. Color and odor come from toxins.

By the way, one thing you might notice with your own kidneys: when you get up first thing in the morning, you have usually not urinated during the whole night. During that time, the kidneys are collecting toxins from the body. So when you first urinate in the morning, your urine should have color in it to show that your kidneys are removing the toxins.

During the day you're drinking liquids, so your urine will not have as much color. This is okay because it's continually flushing out and the water keeps diluting the toxins.

When we see the fabulous design of the body's systems to feed, nourish and cleanse itself, we can only wonder, "Where do we start to rejuvenate the function of these systems?"

CHAPTER THREE

Necessary Changes For Cleansing

Our first step to cleansing is to eliminate the things that are causing an overflow of toxins.

Some of them are: refined salt, refined sugar, caffein, chemicals, hydrogenated fats, food coloring, tobacco, drugs (whether from the street or a doctor), alcohol and preservatives.

Along with this, it's helpful to think about your spiritual level. It's very easy to slide into a rut. It seems like once you hold a grudge against one person, it's easier to hold a grudge against two.

In the same way, once we lie or cheat, it's easier the next time. Sometimes it's easy to think, "Well, I lied about that part. What's the difference if I tell another little lie or not." But lying is not healthy for the body. It really goes against the design of the body, because we have a conscience. Even if it's subconscious, it still wears away at the makeup of our system.

Many people constantly have arguments or disunities with other people, especially in their own families. It's very easy to take it all out on our loved ones and then go outside that circle and be real nice and friendly to everybody else. However, that upsets our system, too. Fits of anger are very detrimental and habit forming.

If you want to get rid of the toxic overload, you

must clean up your lymph system. It's as simple as that. All the previously mentioned negative practices affect and stress the lymph system.

If you start working on your spiritual and physical health at the same time, your mental health will also improve. When you think more clearly, your financial situation usually improves because you not only spend more wisely, you also can earn more easily. It is very difficult to make good decisions, to set goals and even to hold a responsible job when your thinking is impaired by physical ill health.

For a body to gain health and lose weight on a permanent basis, you must be healthy and well-balanced in all areas: mental, physical, spiritual, and financial. In turn this involves cleansing mentally, physically, spiritually and financially. Merely eliminating causes will not correct the total problem. Action must be taken to help the body unload already accumulated waste.

Food as a Form of Cleansing

Proper Food Combining helps the body digest and assimilate nutrients to provide energy to do the cleansing. If you continue to eat foods together that cause poisons and don't digest, you're creating the problem you're trying to eliminate with the cleanse. So you're poisoning yourself as fast as you're releasing poisons. Cleansing and food combining go hand in hand and the body reacts very favorably on such a program. The body loves it. You can actually see faster and faster progress the longer you cleanse and eat properly.

Remember, the body didn't deteriorate overnight, so don't get discouraged if it doesn't recuperate overnight. The body hates fast changes, so it doesn't like it if you try to get well overnight. Go slowly and enjoy it.

Friendly Bacteria — A Food for Cleansing

Many people have heard of yogurt and something about its friendly bacteria. Friendly bacteria help the body cleanse the whole digestive tract.

Here's how it's supposed to work: when food passes from the stomach to the small intestine into the colon, if there's any toxin, the appendix releases a mucus to detoxify it. But, there's so much poison, and since many people don't have their appendix, or the appendix isn't functioning, the bacteria lays there and continues to grow. It is not killed.

A second protection in the digestive tract is supposed to be the friendly bacteria which destroy harmful bacteria. The problem is that if you drink even one cup of coffee, the caffeine will destroy the majority of the friendly bacteria in your colon. Without that friendly bacteria, the harmful bacteria grow wildly.

Take the example of yeast. If you want to make bread rise, you put yeast in it. Because it grows on the bacteria in the air, it causes a gas-type reaction and makes the bread rise.

That's similar to what happens when toxins in the colon mix with harmful bacteria. Yogurt or acidophilus contain the friendly bacteria which will destroy the harmful bacteria.

Scientists know that if you put yogurt in the colon, it causes the colon to manufacture B vitamins. Toxic bacteria grow more rapidly in a colon deficient in B vitamins.

Personal Experience

Years ago when I was very ill, the doctors wanted to do something called exploratory surgery. They decided the best thing to do would be cut me open from the pelvic bone to the rib cage. Then they could take many things out, analyze them, clean them and what wasn't good, they could cut out and then just put everything else back.

So when they told me that, I said, "Doctors, you're looking at a woman who's too chicken to have her ears pierced." I never did have the surgery.

Today when I meet people who I've not seen for 15 to 20 years, they think I've had all kinds of lifts or hormone shots because I look better than I did years ago. When I tell them the improvement is from internal cleansing and Proper Food Combining, they are amazed. My health situation did not happen overnight and it cannot be maintained by an occasional health practice. It's involved years of practice.

But what's so exciting about it is, I look and feel better every year. It puts a lot of fun in your life when you can say that. The fact that I never used drugs or surgery to overcome over 20 major illnesses is a marvelous testimony for the body's ability to cleanse and heal itself.

You can have the same results. So don't be brainwashed into thinking you have to have drugs and you have to have surgery. Take time to think it over. It may be that you will have to have surgery sometime, but learn about your body and how it functions and what preventive measures you can take. Then maybe you'll be able to eliminate potential surgery and drug uses, and improve your health at the same time. And be patient!!!

With all the illnesses I had, none of them depressed me like the obesity and big thighs full of cellulite.

Along with hundreds of clients, I have really appreciated that cleansing does not necessarily eliminate a lot of pounds, but it does eliminate the inches we want eliminated.

Another case involves a young girl called Kim.

Kim used my herbal food, and Proper Food Combining together. Even when she was 100 pounds overweight, her breasts were much too small for the rest of her body.

Kim lost 120 pounds on my program and she lost all those pounds only in her problem areas. She lost 11 inches in each thigh; she lost 12 inches in her hips, but she did not lose even ½ inch in her breasts. At the end of her weight loss, she wore the same size bra cup. She was smaller around the back, because she lost a layer of fat around the back and sides. But the actual bra cup size was the same as before her weight loss.

Many people who lose a pound or two in weight will lose six to 10 inches in their troubled area.

How can that be?

The cleansing only removes toxic weight, not healthy good tissue. So if you cleanse the digestive tract and get it functioning properly, the body goes after the toxins in your legs and arms; your back or buttocks, or wherever they happen to be. Those who have experienced diets where you had to get down to skin and bones before you got rid of the thighs know the value of that.

I've been on many diets and I'd lose from the waist up and I'd still have big thighs. With cleansing, it's the opposite. You keep the good, healthy tissue and you lose the poisons. But you must be patient.

Herbs — Another Food for Cleansing

Most of the world's population use herbs as their major medicine.

For centuries, the Chinese and many other cultures have known that herbs have some type of special power. That power is the energy flow they help provide in the body, so the body can "unplug" itself and get the electricity flowing wherever it is needed to correct a "power failure." Remember that the body is electric. It is a mass of energy. If the electricity is shut off any place in the body it degenerates. (For further information, read *Colon Health* by Norman Walker.) *Each part* of the body has its own electric current. For instance, the kidneys have one wave length and the bladder has another wave length. It's similar to light bulbs: there could be a 40-watt, there could be a 60-watt, and so forth. Not all wattage bulbs will fit in all lamps, or on all currents, but if they do fit, they all give light.

That is how herbs work with the body. Different herbs have "currents" which seem to match different body parts. If the proper herb can be fed that has the same *current* as a disabled body part, the body knows what to take from that food to restart the action needed to correct the problem.

However, just swallowing herbs while continuing to consume garbage food will not correct the problem. It takes a program consistent with the herbal food to help the body maintain the *current* flow.

The body has a specific design in order to heal itself. For example; most people know that if you're having trouble with your eyesight and you eat a lot of carrots, your eyesight will improve. You might wonder why you can't just take a carrot, cut it up and place it in your eye to help your eyesight get better

The design of the body is such that you chew the carrot, digest it, assimilate the nutrients, and then the body knows what it needs out of the carrot for the eyes.

The carrot itself does not heal your eyes, but the nutrients and the vitamins in the carrot can be transformed by the body into a form that can be used by the body. These nutrients are sent to the eyes and the body's use of what's in the carrots helps heal the eyes.

Reversing the Process

With herbs and Proper Food Combining we

reverse the process of deterioration.

We start cleansing and feeding the digestive tract properly. We keep the eliminative organs functioning well. Then the lymph and the blood systems start picking up toxins at the cell level and they start feeding the cells properly.

Pretty soon, you see the pounds and the toxic weight disappear from the whole body. The cleanse doesn't just work on one symptom; it works on the whole body.

Remember that the liver detoxifies, so if it doesn't work, how can you detoxify? The lymph picks up toxins at the cell level, but what if your lymph system or your nodes are so toxic and swollen they can't detoxify? What if you're constipated and you can't get the bowel movements out of the colon? The kidneys cleanse, but what if they don't function properly? The lungs expel poisons, but what if they don't function properly? The skin expels poisons, but what if it isn't functioning properly?

Sometimes when a person starts detoxifying, a serious health problem (which they did not know they had) will manifest itself.

The body has a way of taking the most critical problem and working on it first. For instance, if you were on a liver cleanse and you were involved in an auto wreck and broke your arm, the body would immediately turn all its attention and energy, blood and lymph supply and everything else to that broken arm because it's urgent. The same thing is true when you have surgery. The body goes to the aid of healing the surgery. Everything else becomes secondary.

Your thighs and your legs are outside the digestive system and the digestive system must take care of itself before it can help anything else. We've all heard of cases in which people who were generally unhealthy would break a bone and two years later they would still be walking around with a cast because that bone wouldn't heal properly. If the digestive system is completely toxic, it has nothing to send to help the broken bone.

Internal cleansing does not steal from the body. It does not take anything good from the body. It merely brings about a condition in which the body can rejuvenate itself. Once the kidneys, liver, spleen, pancreas, colon, lymph, blood, and so forth are cleansed and working better, they know how to pick up poisons to flush them out of the body. That is their purpose in the original design of the body. It does not make sense to me to have the very organs removed from your body that were designed to be there to help fight health problems.

If one of the rooms in your house were filthy dirty and it made the rest of the house look bad, would you tear it out of the house? No, you would clean it. You might even paint it, but it would never enter your mind to remove it.

It's the same principle with your body. If that dirty part of the body can be cleansed, clean it and let it remain with the rest of the body to perform its functions.

Cleansing Symptoms

A few people start to cleanse very quickly and when that happens, the poisons release quickly.

People sometimes say to me, "Well, these herbs must be a laxative. As soon as I started taking it, I developed diarrhea."

But the herbs are not being used as a laxative. When the body contains a large amount of toxins that it is trying to release, it sets up a loosening of the bowels in order to flush those poisons out of the body.

If you should experience this, just reduce the amount of herbs to half the amount you were taking. If it is still too strong for you, go back to once a day. For example, take half the amount at breakfast time *only* for one week. The next week, take half at breakfast time and half at lunch. The third week, half with each meal. If you gradually increase the cleanse, the toxins will not release so quickly.

Another thing we have noticed relates to allergies. Allergies are the result of a toxic buildup in the tissue throughout the body. If you start cleansing too fast, it is possible your nose and eyes will secrete mucus as a means of eliminating these loosened toxins. Reduce the use and build up to the recommended level gradually, so that more toxins will be released through the bowel instead of the head area.

The main point is that a few people's bodies release toxins so fast that it feels uncomfortable. We must be able to cleanse and at the same time carry out our normal, daily duties. Don't be in a hurry to accomplish everything overnight. Be patient. Go slowly.

Another possible reaction to the cleanse is an occasional headache and/or nausea. There are two different reasons for this: One, it can be from cleansing. The other could be that you are not drinking enough water.

When the body releases large quantities of toxins, they go through the digestive system to be eliminated. For example toxins might drain from the lymph glands in your throat and your sinus cavities down into the stomach. That could make you a bit nauseated because there will be an excess amount of toxins in the stomach all at once. Drink a glass of water and the nausea is usually gone as soon as you finish drinking the water. The water dilutes the toxins, giving immediate relief.

The same thing is true with a headache. Most people do not realize the importance of water to eliminate headaches. If you have a headache, drink a glass of water. If that doesn't eliminate the headache immediately, try another glass of water in a few minutes. If that doesn't eliminate the headache, it could be from another cause. Headaches are not due to a deficiency of aspirin, so try to correct the problem, not the symptom.

Sometimes people who are changing eating times and no longer snacking on junk food between meals will notice an energy slump. The solution is to drink a glass of water, or a glass of water with a half teaspoon of sugar free dried barley juice. The slump can be from the body using more energy to cleanse, or from concentrated toxins in the digestive tract.

Many people ask, "Is there an appetite suppressant in those herbs? I've noticed since I've been on them I'm not nearly as hungry. In fact, I'm forcing myself to eat."

It's harmful to force yourself to eat if you are truly not hungry. One of the side effects of cleansing (and this is normal) is that you may lose your appetite and become more thirsty.

For example, if you get sick, you don't feel good. Don't you usually find, especially if you have a fever, that you're very thirsty and you really don't care to eat? That is a normal body process. Do what your body wants when you're cleansing. If your body is not hungry, do not feed it. Usually what it needs and wants is more pure liquid.

Sometimes when people use my cleanse they lose the pounds they want to lose, and then think the problem's gone.

That's not so. There is a lot of garbage deep down inside us. I've had people stay on my program for years and they continue to see improvement in all types of health problems which they didn't even think about, or know they had, until they improved.

For instance, a common improvement is skin texture.

People will say, "I have less and less wrinkles all the time." They can't believe that their skin tightens and gets more healthy.

Another thing is an improvement in vision. How many people in this country wear glasses? Yet their vision can, and often does, improve to the point that their lenses need to be changed. Cleansing and Proper Food Combining are a permanent program that continues to benefit overall health.

Sometimes when I say that, people say "Oh, no. I don't want anything I have to continue for a long period of time."

If you have a gallbladder removed, is that for a long period of time?

I can tell you from experience, you will be a lot happier, healthier and thinner if you go on a regular cleansing program than you will be if you go for fad diets, surgery and drugs.

Consider this: if you develop diabetes, you are going to be on a special diet. Why not go on a preventive program now so you never have to be on the diabetic diet?

My Personal Herbal Food – Herbal Trim #1 & #2

When I was very ill and fat, I started using herbs. I experienced some relief from them, but I found that if I put two herbs together, they would do something that they wouldn't do when I used either alone.

For instance, when I learned about cleaning my colon, I discovered that burdock root was helpful because it is also a blood cleanser. I had terrible gout at the time (which is caused by extreme toxins in the blood), so when I started taking burdock, it helped a little bit. But it didn't completely eliminate it.

Then I heard about licorice root and how soothing it is for the digestion, then chickweed, then dandelion, then parsley and saffron.

Over the years this formula evolved through trial and error and *results*. Some people have to adjust the amount they take when they start, but to my knowledge I have never found anyone who could not take the formula. And they get results!

The few people who have had to adjust the formula take smaller amounts when they first start. But if you work with it, you will find that your body will adapt to the cleansing.

Every single organ may not go back to the condition it was five or 10 years ago; but the toxic mucus buildup that is keeping your body from functioning can gradually be eliminated from the body. Thus, the organs will gradually be able to function better.

It is important to remember that the herbs do not heal the body. Only the body can heal itself, and only if it is fed and nourished properly.

My herbal formula will not heal your body. It merely provides a combination of herbs, vitamins and minerals, in their natural form, to help the body use vitamins and minerals to heal itself. Not everyone's body is in the same state of deterioration and not everyone's body is sick in exactly the same location. We all have a different reaction, or rate at which the body recuperates.

One point I'd like to make is this: for the past 25 years my credentials have been based on *results*, first with my own body, then my friends' and neighbors', then with thousands of new friends.

With that principle in mind, let's examine why I use this formula. Keep in mind too that the body's design is to feed and cleanse, feed and cleanse.

The following pages describe the contents of my herbal formula, and which area each herb seems to benefit.

For instance, it has been known for years that echinacea is a food for glands. Salivary glands are located in the mouth. Now if you put food in your mouth and these glands cannot produce saliva, and the saliva doesn't contain ptyalin, which is a digestive enzyme for starch, how are you going to digest it?

Many people tell me that after being on my program they notice, for the first time, they can actually eat a dry food and secrete enough saliva so that that food can start digesting in their mouth.

Licorice is known to help clean the throat. Interestingly enough, professional singers on my program say, "I don't know what it is, but for some reason when I take your herbs I sing better." They can reach notes that they normally can't reach. Or they reach them with a new smoothness. Or they no longer get a sore throat and hoarseness after hours and hours of singing.

Next, the thyroid. Most people know that malfunction of this body part can affect their weight. In fact, many times I'll hear people say, "Well, it's not what I eat. I've always had a sluggish thyroid." But the answer is not necessarily to continue to take drugs or have the thyroid removed. Why not try to rebuild the thyroid with food, with nutrients that the body transforms into energy for the thyroid?

We may find we're deficient in a particular vitamin or mineral and temporarily need to substitute with individual ones. However, there is no better form of food for the body, as far as vitamins and minerals are concerned, than foods in their natural form. That's why, originally, Man ate fruits and vegetation. These had the vitamins and minerals Man needed in a balanced, complete form. Those foods also had roughage and enzymes. No doubt, they also had other things that Man has not even discovered yet that helped the body feed and cleanse itself.

Gradually throughout history, man started substituting for well balanced foods, either with drugs, or with foods that did not have the same nutrients. So our whole body was eventually not getting the energy flow that was needed, or it was getting toxic buildup and mucus that was stopping what energy flow we did have. Since the body's design is so far above Man's comprehension, it only makes sense to eat a whole food and let the body decide what it needs.

Iodine is known to increase thyroid metabolism. Iodine from kelp is in its natural form. It also has many other minerals which are in a balanced form, all of which are needed by the body.

The stomach is where most people seem to notice that they have digestive problems! To help with this, I have used chickweed, black walnut, dandelion (known to help expel poisons), fennel (which helps the body expel toxic gas), licorice root (which helps soothe the stomach), papaya (which aids digestion because of its tremendous amount of digestive enzymes) and vinegar (which is known to reduce putrefaction in the stomach).

When you have a food digesting in the stomach, the body calls extra blood to the digestive area to help in the digestive process. This is one reason why you should never exercise heavily after a meal. It is also one reason why you should not take a hot bath right after eating. These activities keep the blood in the extremities. You don't want that; you want the normal body function, which is for the blood to head toward the stomach to help digestion.

The next digestive organ is the liver. the liver needs iron and this is why I use dandelion. It is known, not for its huge amount of iron, but for the body's ability to assimilate the amount of iron that is in it. I also use fennel which is known to aid the flow of bile and aid the gallbladder.

The pancreas needs zinc. Again, that's why I included dandelion; not for its large amount of zinc, but for the body's ability to use it effectively.

Dandelion also helps feed the spleen. Many people are not very familiar with this organ. It's located a bit underneath your ribs on the left side in the pancreas area.

The spleen has a lot to do with the immune system. Because of so many immune system diseases, we want to make sure that we keep our spleen healthy, because without it, we are missing one of the root foundations of our cleansing system.

For the duodenum or the small intestine, I added black walnut, chickweed, vinegar and fennel. Fennel is known to help the body expel gas.

Many people don't realize that toxins, mucus buildup and gas are in their small intestine area, as well as the colon. If you look on the chart of the digestive system (pages 10 and 11), notice what a large area of the digestive system is covered by the small intestine. People often will start expelling foul-smelling gas when cleansing, because the herbs, by feeding energy to the intestine, help that part of the body to function better and expel old pockets of gas. These old gas pockets can be easily recognized by their extremely foul odor and the heat accompanying the gas. At this point you will learn the true meaning of *Internal Cleansing is an Old Movement.*

Fortunately, this is not an indefinite procedure. Once that gas is out, you will notice it fewer and fewer times the longer that you cleanse. Once it's completely out, it does not tend to build up again as long as you stay on Proper Food Combining and cleansing.

Keep reminding yourself: The only way you can improve the toxic condition of your body is by cleansing and eliminating the causes of the toxins.

Remember, the small intestine is where nutrients go into the body. The lining, or the wall, of the small intestine contains blood capillaries and lymph capillaries which take nutrients back into the system to be used by the entire body. As a result, it is important that this section of the body is cleansed so that it will be able to function properly.

For the large intestine I use burdock, chickweed, dandelion, licorice, parsley, vinegar and saffron. Saffron is known to help expel gas from the bowel or the large colon.

The large intestine is where the final residue of toxins in the body will reside. More and more today, we hear of people developing cancer of the colon. No doubt it is because almost every meal people eat has a toxic buildup which eventually stores in the colon.

The colon needs certain things in order to function well. For instance it needs good nerve tone. So for the nerve tone, I added gotu kola, B^6, vinegar and lecithin.

The colon has muscles which contract, to keep the feces moving toward the rectum. If those muscles don't function properly, and the feces lay there too long, toxins can penetrate right into the tissue of the large colon. So for muscle tone, I added hawthorn berry, B^6, and lecithin.

The colon also needs circulation. Just like the small intestine, the colon has blood and lymph capillaries which feed back to other areas of the body. To feed the colon, I added burdock, echinacea, fennel, hawthorn berry, saffron, and vitamin B^6.

Next, the colon needs biochemical nutrients. This means nutrients that have to do with the life processes, like keeping the whole system of the body going. For this I use kelp, lecithin and B^6.

Let's go on to the lungs. We breath so automatically, we don't even stop and realize what activity must take place for us to breathe.

The lungs are an eliminative organ. We must keep our lungs healthy because of all the poisons constantly being filtered through them. So to help the lungs, I've used chickweed, black walnut, fennel and licorice.

Another eliminative organ is the kidneys. To feed the kidneys I used dandelion, licorice, parsley and lecithin.

Another very important part is the heart. For the heart I added hawthorn berry and licorice. With these two herbs combined, I have seen wonderful results. I've had people tell me that prior to cleansing they have not been able to jog or work out at the spa because of heart problems. They have actually seen such tremendous improvement, they no longer have exercise restrictions.

Again, it was not the herb formula that healed the heart, it was the body's ability to use the nutrients in the herbs.

I have received letters from people, who have been taking heart drugs for as long as 30 years. These people after cleansing, rebuilding their whole system and strengthening the heart muscle, have actually been able to completely eliminate those drugs from their life. When the proper nutrients were consumed, the body was able to convert them into something it could use to heal itself.

Another important function involves the endocrine glands.

Premenstrual syndrome has only been recognized recently by the medical field. Women have recognized it from time immemorial.

As long as 20 years ago, women said to me, "Lee, I don't know what it is, but every since I've been taking those herbs, I'm not hungry for sweets. I don't have the water retention I used to have every month, and I don't get mad and throw fits like I did. Once in a while I feel a little bad, but not at all like I used to."

When you feed the endocrine glands and they are back in balance, you correct the root cause of women's premenstrual syndrome. For this I added hawthorn berry, parsley, chickweed, burdock, kelp, licorice and gotu kola.

The lymph system, as noted above, carries poisons away from the cell.

It *must* function properly. If your lymph system did not function for 24 hours, you would die. In fact, shock is a total body shutdown of the lymph movement in the body. For that I have used echinacea, licorice and hawthorn berry. By the way, echinacea is now recognized worldwide as being beneficial to the immune system in 20 ways. In Germany, over 40 medical products containing echinacea are used by physicians.

The next part of the body is the female organs. For this I have added black walnut, dandelion, fennel, licorice, and saffron.

For depression, I added licorice and hawthorn berry. People who are depressed always have weak adrenal glands. Hawthorn berry is known to be an aid in feeding the adrenal glands.

To reduce nervousness we have found that licorice root and hawthorn berry have been beneficial.

To reduce water retention, I've added burdock, dandelion, fennel, parsley, saffron, B^6 and lecithin. I've been using B^6 for years to reduce water retention, and many doctors are now recommending B^6 and lecithin for women with this problem.

It's also important to keep your blood clean, since it can take nutrients, or poisons, to the cells. For this I have added burdock, chickweed, echinacea and dandelion.

Another problem is anemia. Many people go on a diet and two or three days later they are so weak that they have to eat something. Also, people who have low blood pressure sometimes say, "I have to eat all the time. There's no way I can change my eating habits."

For anemia, I added dandelion and have found that the body really can rejuvenate itself when fed dandelion. I have also found that any almost any green leaf food seems to have something the body can use for anemia.

Herbal Formula — Contents and Effects

Organ or Symptom	Beneficial Herb
Mouth	Echinacea
Throat	Licorice
Thyroid	Kelp
Stomach	Chickweed, black walnut, dandelion, fennel, licorice, root, papaya, vinegar
Liver	Dandelion, fennel
Gallbladder	Fennel
Pancreas	Dandelion (zinc)
Spleen	Dandelion
Small Intestine	Black walnut, chickweed, vinegar and fennel

Organ or Symptom	Beneficial Herb
Large Intestine	Burdock, Chickweed, dandelion, licorice, parsley, vinegar and saffron
Nerve Tone	Gotu kola, B^6, vinegar, lecithin
Colon muscles	Hawthorne berry, B^6, lecithin
Colon circulation	Burdock, echinacea, fennel, hawthorne berry, saffron, B^6
Colon nutrients	Kelp, lecithin, B^6
Lungs	Chickweed, black walnut, fennel, licorice
Kidneys	Dandelion, licorice, parsley, lecithin
Heart	Hawthorne berry, licorice
Endocrine Glands (and P.M.S.)	Hawthorne berry, parsley, chickweed, burdock, kelp, licorice, gotu kola
Lymph	Echinacea, licorice, hawthorne berry
Female organs	Black walnut, dandelion, fennel, licorice, saffron
Depression	Licorice root, hawthorne berry
Adrenal Glands	Hawthorne berry
Nervousness	Licorice root, hawthorne berry
Water Retention	Burdock, dandelion, fennel, parsley, saffron, B^6, lecithin
Blood Cleansing	Burdock, chickweed, echinacea, dandelion
Anemia	Dandelion, green leafed food

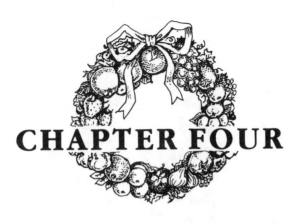

Other Forms of Internal Cleansing

Internal cleansing can be greatly facilitated when you combine cleansing and Proper Food Combining with other cleansing techniques, exercise, and improvement of mental attitudes. In this chapter, I will discuss each of these activities and their effects on overall health in some detail.

Exercise: A Program for *You*

People often ask me about exercise. The lymph system is moved by two methods; deep breathing and massage. Deep breathing during exercise increases the lymph movement by tenfold. Therefore, it is important for you to get exercise, but it must be exercise that will not harm you more than it helps you.

Many people are not well enough to exercise. If a body has an extreme toxic buildup, it also means that the muscles, tendons and other body parts are infected with toxic buildup. That means they are not supple; they do not "give" or flex properly. If such a person suddenly starts jogging on hard cement and doing exercises during which he or she stresses and strains, or pulls and lifts weights, damage to these sick muscles and tendons is a good possibility.

Doctors report that at one time a large increase in business was from people who were jogging and putting stress on their body which it was not well enough to handle.

If you do want to start an exercise program, start with things you enjoy doing. For instance, if you like to swim, swim. You don't have to lift weights and look macho to get the benefit from swimming. You will breathe more deeply. You'll get the lymph moving. You'll move muscles and you'll do it in the water where you are less likely to strain them.

Bicycle riding is another option. Remember, though, when you're tired, quit riding. Don't go for a 10-mile trip the first time you ride. I know a man who did that once. He rode three miles out into the country and had to call his wife to have her pick him up in order to get back.

Don't feel you have to be an Olympic potential in order to do exercise. Anything you do that makes you breathe heavier, or move muscles that you don't ordinarily move, is a good exercise for you.

I personally love to roller skate and sing. I also like to dance and sing, but I don't go to smoky bars, so I go to the roller rink. I skate for three hours, and during that time, I think about anything and everything — sometimes about business. My best business ideas have come while I was roller skating. But I don't skate to become a professional roller skater. I skate to use the muscles in my legs I don't ordinarily use. I perspire. I get my lymph moving and I love the music and the skate dancing.

I come out so refreshed, not only physically, but mentally, and I've improved the circulation of blood and lymph through my body, which is going to help cleanse tissue.

Walking is by far the best exercise with which to start. But it is important to walk regularly. It's okay to walk in the rain, or the snow, the sunshine or whatever weather condition prevails. But do walk every day. In fact, try to take a brisk 30-minute walk every day. Swing your arms a little. It helps improve your breathing and your circulation.

I try to walk an hour every day. But I don't run-walk; I walk. I walk at a nice pace, so I can notice the flowers and the trees and improve my mental attitude. I see things going on in the neighborhood that I would never know were happening unless I was out for a walk. Now, I realize some neighborhoods are too dangerous to walk. So, you may have to walk around your house, around your own block, around your apartment — but *walk*.

Whatever exercise you do, make sure you are enjoying it.

Don't force yourself and say, "Oh, it's Monday night. I've worked all day and now I have to go to the spa tonight." It may be all over right there, because your body won't be happy. If it's a drudgery, it will show up in your mind and your muscles when you go to work out at the spa.

It's true that sometimes you think you're too tired and if you exercise anyway you'll feel good after you do it. If that happens to you and you can overcome that resistance, fine. The point is, exercise should be constructive, not destructive.

The Mini-Trampoline — One exercise that has benefited even paralyzed people is using a mini-trampoline.

You can use a little trampoline and benefit by moving the lymph, learning breathing exercises, and improving your cardiovascular system.

The following is just one example of how to use the mini-trampoline:

First of all, before you start doing anything, breathe deeply a few times to make sure you're healthy enough to tolerate deep breathing. Most of us breathe shallowly and we never get a good supply of oxygen to the brain. So when we start doing something that makes us breathe deeply, we take a few breaths and we're light-headed. I don't want you to fall off the trampoline, so take a few deep breaths first. If you don't get dizzy from it, it's okay to proceed. If you get dizzy do some more deep breathing for a while before you get on the trampoline.

Next, stand on the trampoline and spread your legs to get a good balance. Now, lift up your right heel and put it down. Next lift up your left heel and put it down. Don't pick up your whole foot, just the heel. Now get a little rhythm going. It's right heel up, left heel up; right heel up, left heel up.

Try to do that for about one minute. Keep doing it and at the same time, *if you're strong enough,* take a deep breath. If you get dizzy, stop for a few minutes and just stand still.

By using x-rays, it's been proven that the lungs act like a suction pump and when you suck air deeply into your lungs, it moves the lymph.

When I tell this to some people, they really get carried away.

They say, "Well, if breathing deeply does that, shouldn't I run and sweat and really breathe heavy to get that lymph moving?"

The answer is "Yes, if you are healthy enough." But you probably aren't, so just be patient. Back up a little bit and go slowly. Start working with your trampoline four to five times daily, four to five minutes at a time.

Even before the five minutes are up, some people get a cramp in the calf. Just stop until it goes away, get back on your trampoline and do it again for a few minutes.

Your goal is eventually to be able to use the

trampoline for hours without getting tired, without feeling any pull or muscles in your legs, and at the same time being able to breathe deeply. This is not hard to do. It can be done right in your home, in bad weather, and in dangerous neighborhoods. But it is effective, so you must gradually work into it.

I've bounced for five hours without stopping. I had more energy when I stopped than when I started!

I have had marvelous success from using the mini-trampoline with paralyzed people, with children, with middle-aged people and with people with allergies. This is because it gets that lymph moving and really helps the system detoxify.

The Slant Board — It is incredible all the health benefits that come with merely laying down on a slant board. With gravity pulling everything down 24 hours per day, 15 minutes on the slant board performs miracles.

While on the slant board, blood flows to the top of the head. Prolapsed organs have a chance to relax from the stress, and the muscles of those organs receive a new blood supply, helping them rebuild themselves.

Many people make their own slant board using just a sheet of plywood with a pad on it. Elevate one end 17 to 24 inches off the floor and lie on it with your feet at the elevated end. Nothing to it!!

When you first use the board, you will feel blood rush to your head. If it is too much pressure for you, simply stand up slowly and in a little while try it again. It won't take long until you will easily be able to lie there the whole 15 minutes.

This is such a relaxing form of internal cleansing that often times I fall asleep for 30 to 40 minutes.

If you would like company during your workout, my exercise video shares 15 minutes of easy to do exercises on the mini-trampoline and 15 minutes on the slant board – see order form "Exercise Video".

More Vigorous Exercise — Many people are now involved in weight lifting. They want that muscular look and more vigorous exercise.

If you get cellulite connected to muscle, it takes twice as long to get that cellulite off as it does when it's not in a muscle.

So the process to use is: first cleanse and detoxify. At the same time use Proper Food Combining so you can strengthen yourself. Then start some mild exercise, such as walking, or using the mini-trampoline. Then, after your body is really in shape, you can go on to these stronger efforts if you want.

I know some people think "I'm healthy enough. I work hard every day. I'm in good shape; I am sure I can handle some good workouts."

From personal experience I can tell you that you can do a lot of damage. Years ago I had a twisted pelvis, of which I was unaware.

I started going to a well-known workout gym. I was fat from the waist down, and I had the usual idea that what I needed was some strong exercise after sitting at a desk all day. In fact, my doctor told me that.

My pelvis was ¼ inch higher on the right side and 1½ inches further forward on the right side. That continual strain pulled my spine out of alignment and pulled all the muscles that held my colon. That's why my colon finally collapsed.

At that gym, I did all the exercise possible to decrease my big thighs. But instead my legs started getting bigger. Not only did my legs get bigger, but I started having terrible headaches and backaches.

You see, the pelvis was already in trouble and then I started doing leg lifts which pulled it more and more out of place, and it only made the problem worse.

The exercise we need is exercise that helps the body cleanse, first of all. Then worry about muscles later. We must detoxify first.

Internal Bathing

Drinking a lot of plain water is one method of bathing the whole digestive tract.

Nothing substitutes for water. You should, and can, drink water anytime except within 15 minutes before eating and two hours after eating. Your total water consumption per day should be approximately 64 oz. for a five foot tall person. Adjust per size.

There is so much controversy over water today as to whether to drink steam distilled, or reverse osmosis water.

I recommend that you investigate various water purifiers and choose the one which fits your local area and your needs. Here's why: I was going to buy a water purifier in Washington. I took some water from Arizona to Washington with me to have it tested to make sure the machine would purify my water. The Arizona water tested so full of chemicals that the machine would not handle it. The machine could handle Washington water, but not Arizona water.

Personally, I still think steam distilled (if it really is steam distilled) is the best. The problem is knowing for sure if it is actually pure steam distilled.

Steam distilled water is *very* beneficial in washing accumulated minerals from the body. I have had many experiences with arthritic clients and by only changing to steam distilled water they have experienced improvement. Minerals which have become part of the cell structure do not wash out with water. If you have consumed minerals which have not become part of the cell structure, they are "deposits" and these "deposits" settle especially in joints throughout the body. Experience has shown these are the minerals steam distilled water washes from the body.

Three additional methods of bathing the digestive tract are:

      (1) using an enema bottle
      (2) using a colonic 'board'
      (3) using a professional colonic.

I have experienced all three methods.

The Enema Bottle — Of course, I used enemas for years because I could not afford any other treatment. Even though I was not educated on enemas, I realized the benefit I gained from what I did. One problem I consistently see with enemas is that most people try to rush them. This is no doubt due to the fact you must get on and off the toilet quite often if you spend much time with it. If you cannot afford any method besides an enema, plan to spend 30 to 40 minutes to fill the water bag and absorb and release the water through your rectum, over and over.

An enema bottle can be purchased at most drug stores. It looks like a one-quart hot water bottle with a long tube attached.

The enema bottle tube is placed in the rectum and, for the sake of comfort, some sort of lubrication should be used when inserting the tube. I always lie flat on the floor with a large towel under me. Some people sit in their bathtub and I recently heard of a person who just sat on the toilet.

The enema bottle should be hung high enough above you so that the water will flow freely. (If you lie on the floor it works perfectly to hang the bottle on a door knob.)

As the water runs in, you will feel an urge to defecate. Best results come if you can hold the water a few minutes, but do not become uncomfortable.

The Colonic Board is a flat board which is very convenient because it has an opening on one end which is placed over the toilet. You merely lie on the board and the water runs in and out of you without you having to get up and down on the toilet.

The water container used with the colonic board is a four-gallon bucket with a tube attached similar to the one with an enema bottle. You insert the tube into the rectum and leave it while you are on the board. The rectum muscles hold the tube in the rectum even while you are releasing water.

I have found the colonic board to be much more comfortable and much more effective than enemas or the machine colonics. I like to do my own analyzing of what releases from my body and the home colonic board gives me that option. I also like receiving all the treatment possible in the privacy of my own home. Any place "clinical" automatically takes away from the comfort of a loving home. Colonic boards can usually be purchased at national health conventions, or check with your local health food store. Or, send a self-addressed stamped envelope to my office.

The Professional Colonic is an option some people prefer. Find a person who does more than just inject a lot of water into your intestine. Find one who massages the colon area and the nerve endings in the feet or along the spine. Some use acidophilus or yogurt in the water; or they'll have you take some acidophilus orally when the colonic is completed.

It is very important that the colonic office be immaculately clean. Be sure to examine both the operator's qualifications and the facility before treatment.

Colonics can be a marvelous treatment when combined with cleansing, especially if fasting to release toxins. If you have a colonic once a day, all that water helps flush out those released toxins. Thus, they don't lay there and seep through the lymph and blood system back into the body.

The number of internal baths, and when you have them, should be your decision. You are the only one who knows if you feel like you need one. Most people prefer the evening because they seem to sleep better. Also, it keeps the waste from lying in the colon all night.

People who are fasting find an internal bath necessary every day they are on the fast. And persons fasting more that three days find it necessary to bathe internally every time they have a mood that is anything but happy. Yes, your brain is affected too!

I've heard many pros and cons on enemas and colonics. I'm not advising you one way or another, but these thoughts might help you decide.

At one time some people from another country lived next to me and they were always telling me about enemas. I was very young and I'd never heard of enemas. When they described to me what they would do, I thought, "Boy, these people are really weird. Anybody who would put a tube up their rectum and flush quarts and quarts of water into themselves and do all the rest that goes with that has to be insane."

Then one day I found out that they were both in their 90s. I had thought at the most they were 50. I did a double-take and said, "Why do you look so young?"

They said, "Because we eat lots of yogurt and we take enemas."

I didn't take that to heart much, although I did start eating yogurt. But I didn't know how to do enemas.

A few years later I was watching a television program about how so many animals give themselves enemas. I was amazed, because it was the same principle that my neighbors had described to me and it surprised me enough to investigate the matter.

I started experimenting and learning how to do enemas. It amazed me when I learned how few people know how to give themselves enemas. I guess it's because it's a subject about which we never talk. We're never taught as a child how to do it. And yet in countries all over the world, such internal bathing is a common health practice.

Examining the Old Movement — Things seem to come naturally to us if we learn them from infancy. That's how it is with examining your own bowel movement. The problem is that we don't learn to do this from infancy and, as adults, we are very squeamish about doing such a thing.

As parents you may remember checking your baby's diaper. What were you looking for? You were checking to see how they were functioning *internally*.

As adults, we have to use another method to retain our feces so that we can examine them. This is one way you could do it.

Find a pasta strainer that has a wire screen (like that used in screen doors, only finer). This strainer should be approximately eight inches across at the widest part and should have a handle.

Then install it in your toilet. Lift the toilet lid, next lift the ring (the part you sit on) and facing the toilet put your strainer directly down in the water. The handle should not get in the water, just the screen. Then put the toilet ring back down.

When you go to the bathroom, you merely sit down on the toilet, pass your bowel movement, and the screen will catch it. The first few times you may be a bit squeamish, but after that you find yourself looking forward to going to the bathroom.

In order to review the waste, you merely shake the handle of the strainer. Current feces will go through the screen, but the old rubber, mucus, stones, etc. will remain inside the screen. They cannot get through the screen. This makes it very easy for you to then lift the strainer out of the water and using a spoon (it does not have to be a silver spoon!) you merely check through to see what came out. When you're done put the strainer back in the toilet water, and rinse it and flush the waste away. Easy!!!!

If you should find anything in the screen that you want to save just pick it out, rinse it and unless it is kidney stones, you must freeze it or put it in formaldehyde.

When I passed my 3½-foot-long piece of rubber, I got so excited I forgot and flushed it down the toilet. Be a little wiser if you find something that great! Also, to show you how toxic that waste is . . . I left the bathroom for approximately 30 minutes and when I went back in the odor was so extremely horrible I could not stand it. Better down the toilet than in you!!!

Sometimes when people are cleansing and I start to question them to see if they are passing the "old movement," they say, "No, I haven't noticed anything." They also haven't been straining or checking thoroughly. They merely look in the water and that is not enough.

Most people's bowel movements sink, so if you do not have a strainer, use a spoon to stir the water. That way the feces will come up where you can see it.

If you pass kidney stones you will not be able to find them without a strainer, because they are too small. I have had clients pass one-half cup full of kidney stones, and they didn't even know they had them until they saw them in the strainer. Do not presume you don't have them; presume you do, and then if you don't, all the better.

There is usually no pain when you pass these old

movements. At the most you may experience a gas pocket passing, but you are probably passing those most of the time already. If you have ever passed a kidney stone, or gallstone, without cleansing, you know how uncomfortable that can be. It is much better to get them out with cleansing *before* they move on their own.

One thing you will notice in your self-examinations is that if you eat a lot of meat, which is a dead food, your bowel movements will stink all the time. There's no way you can get around it. Most vegetarians do not have smelly bowel movements, except the old ones that move out during cleansing. The by-products from digesting meat leave heavy toxins in the digestive tract and of course, this creates odor.

Identifying A Normal Bowel Movement — The colon is 2½ inches in circumference and approximately five feet long. I want to explain to you how you can identify a normal bowel movement.

A normal bowel movement will be approximately 2½ inches around, the same as the colon. It will be dark in color because residue from the liver bile that breaks down red blood cells is dark in color. The healthy bowel movement will float on the top of the water and it will usually be long.

A floating bowel movement shows you have good roughage, mucus, friendly bacteria and other normal contents. If it is long, your colon is cleaning and functioning fairly well.

Everyday short, sinking bowel movements can mean many problems throughout the whole digestive tract. However, when you are cleansing you may pass some of these because the colon is emptying them from old pockets. The cleansing bowel movements will be accompanied by a uniquely horrible odor. You won't have any problem identifying the old movements!!!

Cleansing vs. More Dramatic Treatment — One caution: there is a time to cleanse and a time for more drastic measures, such as drugs and surgery.

Cleansing is a preventive measure to reduce your chances of needing drugs or surgery for things that have accrued over a long period. That is not the same as an accident or an injury. If you are injured and in an ambulance on the way to a hospital, do not tell the paramedics that you want to go home and cleanse.

One thing you might consider, though, is that the better your health is, the better your chances of survival and healing if you should become injured.

Rest and Sleep

Another method the body uses for internal cleansing is rest and sleep.

Sleep helps the body to recuperate physically and mentally. Sleep renews the body's energy, gives it a psychological lift and prepares the person to work with greater enthusiasm.

Research has shown that sleep puts the body and mind on a holding pattern, allowing the body to catch up with the fatigue that has accumulated during waking hours. As we sleep, the self-healing mechanisms work on repairing whatever has been damaged or worn out.

When deprived of sleep for long periods, we discover that even the simplest of tasks begin to seem stressful. We become irritable and short-tempered. Our appetites become abnormal. We are mentally distracted, make mistakes, and we are unable to concentrate. Our mental and emotional lives suffer, and our bodies suffer, because we become more susceptible to diseases of all kinds.

Scientists don't yet understand all the healing properties of sleep, but research has shown that some systems are at work during sleep. During sleep new cells in the mucosal tissue of our mouths, needed to replace cells damaged by trauma, infection, and age, are produced much more rapidly than in our waking hours.

As we sleep our arterial blood pressure drops, our pulse rate decreases, our skin vessels dilate, and muscles throughout our bodies become completely relaxed. Activity within our nervous system slows.

Some research has shown that six hours of sleep when the stomach is empty is equal in restfulness to eight hours with an overloaded stomach. Do not eat shortly before going to bed.

I have found that if anyone is cleansing and they feel any type of tiredness, it is usually the body trying to tell them to get more rest.

With all of this in mind, doesn't it seem reasonable that if a person is serious about improving his or her health, sufficient rest and sleep is a wonderful part of the internal cleansing?

For further information to obtain a Colonic Board or Lee's Herbal Formula, call (602) 863-2715.

CHAPTER FIVE

Questions About Cleansing

This chapter includes some frequently asked questions about cleansing. If your question is not answered, feel free to write me, enclosing a self-addressed, stamped envelope.

Question: How long did it take you to lose your 50 pounds of waste?

Lee: I almost hesitate to answer that because I was so ill, and because so few of my organs functioned properly, I could not take the toxic weight off until the organs started functioning properly again.

I did lose some weight for a while, for instance, when I first started cleansing my colon. At that time I didn't know my kidneys weren't functioning properly. I had huge thighs, which I now know are one symptom of improperly cleansing kidneys. So until I cleansed the kidneys, I could not eliminate the rest of the excess weight.

This didn't happen overnight. It took 10 years before my health was *close* to where it should be. Today, it would probably not take so long because there is more knowledge available on self-care and body cleansing.

So how long it takes you to lose the pounds is not the important thing; the important thing is that you are constantly cleansing so your organs can eventually function better. Then your body and proper diet will take care of the excess weight.

Question: How much will I lose?

Lee: It is not how many pounds you lose that's important, it's how much poison you eliminate.

The uppermost thought should be "How can I keep cleansing? Don't let me put anything in my mouth that will cause a poison buildup." You will not only have pound loss, you will also have inch loss without it resulting in flabby skin.

I'm not saying that if you're 50 pounds overweight, it's not important that you take those 50 pounds off. What I am saying is that mentally it helps to adjust your thinking — not toward pounds lost, but to the actual cleansing achieved. For one thing, if you are very aware of not taking toxins into your body and at the same time cleansing it, you will get at the root of the problem.

People who are using the Proper Food Combining and my herbal formula together are losing weight, inches, and toxins at a phenomenal rate, much faster than they ever have before, even when previously on a starvation program. Many call me and tell me they are eating three times the amount of food and still dropping 10, 20, and 30 pounds a month.

These are the results possible when people do not put garbage into their mouth anymore. They have stopped consuming large amounts of alcohol. They have started doing exercise that helps the eliminative organs work and they are faithfully taking herbs. As a result they see phenomenal health benefits along with weight loss.

A woman called me who had lost only two pounds during the first two weeks. But she had lost nine inches at the waist. She could wear clothes that she hadn't worn for 10 or 20 years. She said she passed gas so constantly during the initial cleansing that she felt like a walking popcorn popper.

What was causing her waistline to protrude those extra nine inches was not a thick layer of fat. She could have cut her calories down to almost nothing and try to burn off fat, but that was not the problem. The problem was gas and toxic buildup in the digestive tract. So when she started passing all the gas, it relieved the pressure from the organs, which were malfunctioning because of the stress on them. As that gas was released, her organs started functioning better.

I've always said, "I don't care if I weigh 300 pounds as long as I continue to wear size 3 slacks." We all know that's impossible, but the point is . . . it's not always pound loss that is most important. The most important thing is how much toxin you eliminate.

People often say to me, "I have to lose 20 pounds. I've never fit into size 7 or 8 or 9 (or whatever) unless I get down to a certain poundage."

Yet they'll cleanse, lose only 10 pounds, and find they're fitting into the clothes size they want to be. That is because they lost the weight and the inches only where the problem was.

Question: I'm on medication. Can I take the herbs with my medication?

Lee: Yes, but I want to point out that medication can slow down the effectiveness of herbs. Often that is because drugs are detrimental to the body. It doesn't matter why you are using them, or whether you get them from your doctor or on the street. They only pacify a problem; they do not correct it.

However, I do *not* encourage anyone who is on medication to just stop taking it. Even if it should happen that you no longer need the medication, the body gets addicted to any drug and depends on it. Also, any time you stop taking a drug, it should be a gradual process unless the circumstances are unusual. And you are the only one who really knows at what pace you may decrease medication. Even your doctor cannot tell you because he doesn't know how you feel.

As an example, if you're on thyroid medication and you decide to decrease your intake only you know when you start to feel a difference. The doctor can't tell you. "If you cut that in half, in three days you're not going to feel as well as you do now." You're the only one who will know. Nonetheless, if you are going to try to get off medication, consult your doctor, tell him what you're going to do.

Question: How long should I take the herbal formula?

Lee: Only as long as you want to improve your health and stay thin.

I don't actually know that there's any limit. I have had people taking it for years. They continue to feel better. They continue to look younger. Their skin condition continues to be more healthful-looking. They wouldn't think of stopping.

Question: Will I get flabby?"

Lee: I have not found this to be a problem, even with large and rapid weight losses.

When you use the Proper Food Combining with cleansing, you do not count calories or carbohydrates and in most instances, you are actually eating more food than you previously did. So you are getting plenty of nourishment from your diet. The body converts this nourishment into food for the skin, as well as for the rest of the body. Therefore you would not normally have the flabby skin or the drawn-out look that many people get when they lose weight too rapidly by decreasing calories.

Question: Will I lose all over my body?

Lee: If you have toxins all over your body, you will lose weight all over your body. Many women appreciate this program because most women do not have cellulite in their breasts. They may have cysts or tumors, but they don't have cellulite. So when they use this program, they do not lose good breast tissue.

I have had clients who had fibroid cysts in their breasts. When the cysts dissolved, their breasts became smaller as far as filling out the cup, but the actual breasts were not smaller. The only reduction in size was from the elimination of the cysts.

Question: Should I take the herbal formula three times a day, when I don't eat three times a day?

Lee: Maneuver your own schedule to fit in the cleanse. You may cleanse rapidly enough so that you need only take the herbs twice a day when you eat your meals. But for the average person, the recommended dosage is three times a day.

If you skip a meal you should still take the herbs. If you're skipping lunch take formula number 1 at 12 o'clock noon, for example. Then, at 12:30 or 12:45 take formula number 2 as though you had a meal in between.

Question: Should I drink diet sodas to lose weight?

Lee: Advertisers use great sales pitches: There are no calories, or there is only one calorie, and a girl comes out of a swimming pool who looks just like we've always dreamed we could look.

It's true that diet sodas have almost no calories, but they also are probably the most fattening food or drink on the market.

To begin with, they're chemicals. Every client I have had who used diet sodas over a period of time, (and for that matter, even regular sodas) had kidney problems. Most of them didn't even know they had kidney problems until they started to cleanse.

When the kidneys do not function properly, putrid urine deposits remain in the body. Remember if you have a specific, critical problem the whole body makes sacrifices to help eliminate the problem. That's what happens when people go on my herbal formula cleansing program.

Let's say a person goes on the program and loses approximately 10 pounds. Then all of a sudden the weight loss stops and they can't lose any more weight, no matter what they do. If they try my deeper kidney cleanse, it brings about wonderful results. Often they lose as much as 10 pounds during the three-day cleanse and from that time on, their weight loss continues.

There are two more things that diet sodas do. They destroy the vitamin C in your body. In addition, the artificial sweeteners in them are known to cause liver tumors.

This is the experience of a woman who drank two quarts of diet sodas every day for years. She only ate 500 calories a day and she never ate more than 30 carbohydrates per day. This woman had never been able to lay in bed more than six hours at a time without developing terrible backaches.

After a month on my herbal formula her weight loss stopped and no matter what she did, she couldn't lose another pound. She did not know she had kidney problems until it became apparent while cleansing. She did my kidney cleanse for three days. As a result, she passed urine so toxic she blistered her whole private area down to the knees.

After that cleanse, for the first time in her life, she could lay in bed without getting a backache. She lost seven pounds in three days, even though her carbohydrate count was probably in the hundreds. She then went back on my herbal formula for a month and lost more weight.

Two months later, she did the kidney cleanse again and the second cleanse brought out more poisons. The urine was almost chocolate brown, but there was no more blistering of the skin. She does the kidney cleanse every six months and she no longer has a weight problem. She no longer has kidney problems. She no longer drinks diet sodas!

I always encourage everyone to proceed slowly.

Had I known this woman was blistering from the urine toxins, I would have had her stop after just one day on the cleanse, then do it again for one day at a time until some of those toxins were released. But this woman was so determined to lose weight that she suffered through it all and it turned out okay.

However, if you start a cleanse and you have a severe reaction because of cleansing too fast, stop and wait a few days, or a few weeks, and try again. Remember the point is you are getting better every day, so it doesn't have to be done overnight. You have time.

Question: What about Nutra-Sweet, or Aspertame?

Lee: It's another artificial sweetener and we've already discussed the value of artificial sweeteners. The body just simply does not flourish on artificial *anything*.

However, an additional point is this. The previous artificial sweeteners discussed damage mainly the kidneys and the bladder. In fact, some research shows that people who drink diet sodas stand a 60 percent higher chance of having cancer of the bladder than people who don't.

But with Aspertame there is now strong suspicion of brain interference. It may not bother the kidneys and the bladder, but it may interfere with the electrical currents in your brain. Scientists have found, especially with fetuses in the womb, that there is a negative effect on the baby.

I've had people relate experiences where they lost many mental faculties while using Aspertame and only the discontinuance of its use helped relieve the problem. It's artificial and the design of the body was never intended to handle anything artificial. If you need to sweeten things, you're probably not getting enough fruit. Increase — double, triple, quadruple — your fruit consumption and you'll see you don't have the same hunger for sweets.

Question: Will your herbal formula help clean out that hard rubber from the colon?

Lee: Yes, in most cases. But you have to be patient and keep using it. There are cleanses that would clean that rubber out in no time, but you would be in bed 24 hours a day for a few weeks. Most people don't have time for that.

My herbal formula is designed so you can take it every day and the body cleans slowly and mildly enough that you don't get ill. You can still do your housework, you can hold a job, and you can have a social life.

If you stir up too many poisons too fast, you will become ill because your body can't dispose of it fast enough. So just take it slowly, continue to use it, and you will find by checking your bowel movements that pieces of rubber will come out.

Question: What about fasting?

Lee: If you're a person who has used a lot of drugs, no matter what kind, you should not fast for long periods of time. The reason is that regardless of what you've been told, a residue of those drugs remains at the cellular level. If you start fasting and cleansing rapidly, you can release too many of those drugs at one time and you can actually overdose, or have a drug reaction.

Do not start a program by fasting. You must be well enough to fast. Do some mild cleansing and food combining first.

Question: Should I use salt?

Lee: I thought that everybody had realized how dangerous salt is for your health. I'm not talking about sodium, the natural kind that is in fruits and vegetables. I'm talking about white, refined salt.

It causes water retention and high blood pressure. It interferes with normal body function. Remember the sodium-potassium pump at the cell level we described earlier? It interferes with that and keeps it from working properly. It also damages your kidneys.

If you crave salt or sugar, it is a sign of illness in the body. Both refined sugar and refined salt act as drugs in the body. They both distort your taste buds.

Question: Can children use the herbal formula?

Lee: Yes, children as young as two years old, 11 years old, 13 years old, and many different ages have used it.

One child aged 2½ years had been paralyzed in an auto wreck. Her bowels never moved on their own after her injury until they started giving her small bits of the powder from my herbal formula.

If you're going to give it to your children, adjust the dosage according to their age and size. Some children at 13 are as large in body as I am, but you must remember their body will work faster because it's younger. So start them on a small amount, watch their bowel movements and then increase the amount of the formula according to what you think they need to start moving out the toxins.

You will be amazed at the old movements which

will come out of your children's bodies. I have many clients who put their children on the herbs during summer school vacation and they also do Proper Food Combining along with it. Every one of them says that it improves the mental disposition of the children and the parents.

If your child is overweight, you may want to nip that problem in the bud. Also, many children who have acne have benefited from the herbs because they help clean those toxins out and regulate body functions.

Question: Will your my herbal formula help constipation?

Lee: I would say from all the wonderful reports we receive that it has helped many people eliminate constipation. And, if you want to eat a fruit along with the program to help either diarrhea or constipation, bananas are known to help correct both.

As I mentioned before, about the only time a person on my herbs will experience constipation is if they've been eating large volumes of food and the colon muscle has not been working for so long that they need that volume to keep shoving the food through. Temporarily, you might increase the amount of herbs. You can double whatever dosage you're using until the bowels are loosened and they're back to normal. Then cut back to your regular dosage.

I'd like to relate an experience of a boy who was paralyzed, when he was 15 years old.

For 2½ years he did not have a bowel movement on his own. The nurses would have to go up through the rectum surgically and remove the bowel movements. Suppositories and enemas would not work because he didn't have any muscular activity to eject it.

His massage therapist started him on my herbal formula. On the fifth day of taking it, he had a bowel movement on his own.

What was interesting to me was that his physical therapist, who is legally blind, said that before using the herbs she could feel a slight temporary improvement but as soon as she stopped massaging the muscles the tissue would re-tighten.

Almost immediately after using the herbs, she said she could feel the difference in what happened with that tissue. The tissue would hold and stay more relaxed after she had massaged it.

This boy continues to have treatments. He's at the point now where he rocks in a rocking chair because the movement helps move the lymph that takes toxins away from those dead muscles and it acts as an electric pump for him. His whole body is starting to be rejuvenated.

Question: If I start doing enemas or colonics, will I become dependent on them?

Lee: Not if you are practicing other health habits. Occasionally, I meet a person who felt if they used enemas they could then eat and drink whatever they wanted. They were thus using the enemas as a crutch. Do not allow that to happen. If you use enemas and/or colonics with a good total program as outlined in this book, you will find that you will have *more* bowel movements than you had prior to using the internal bathing.

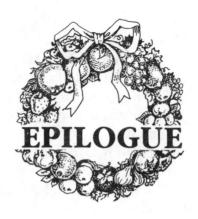

EPILOGUE

It's Up To You

The main things you want to keep in your mind are:

1. Do not put poisons into your body;
2. Eliminate the ones that are there already.

As the design of all life on earth shows, this two-fold activity is a must in order to maintain life. The best way I know to do that is internal cleansing and Proper Food Combining.

I have studied cleansing and diet for over 20 years and I use this cleansing program and Proper Food Combining.

I have stayed with this program because of the RESULTS thousands have experienced. I've had significant health improvement because I have applied exactly what I teach in my seminars and what I have written in this book.

Good health to you, in body, in mind, and in spirit.

Testimonial Letters

I have received letters from people about their experiences with my herbal formula and Proper Food Combining. These are not exceptional cases, but I want you to know what other people have experienced.

Their results are typical of what can happen to you on this cleansing, nourishing program.

In December of 1984 a woman had been on the herbal cleanse for 21 days. She wrote:

> I've been on the herbal formula since December 3, and have lost 10 pounds and 8 inches in my waist. Imagine that, 10 pounds but 8 inches. Now you look at 8 inches on a rule; I mean, that's a lot to lose around the waist, too, right? And, I have lost two inches in my hips. I am delighted.

Here's another:

> I wanted to thank you again for our talk the other day and to tell you how much your herbal formula has changed my life.
>
> I am 44 years old and until mid-April of this year, (1984) was looking and feeling every year of my age and then some. I found that dessert for every meal was a bad case of indigestion followed by hours of lower intestinal distress. In addition, I was 20 pounds heavier than I cared to admit. Just as I was beginning to think I was having some dread disease, my sister attended your seminar and brought me home your Proper Food Combining chart and your wonderful tape.
>
> Incredibly, I not only felt 100 percent better within one week, but by the first week in May, I was wearing my size 10 clothes again. I am bombarded with compliments about my appearance, but what I really appreciate is the way I feel.

The point that is important here is the way she feels. The pound loss and the inch loss came automatically as she was cleansing with herbs and Proper Food Combining.

Here's a letter from another woman:

> I have been a fan of many beautiful, famous people in my life and yet I've never taken the time to write a fan letter. This is my first.
>
> The morning I heard your lecture was my lucky day. Everything you touched on seemed to be what I was experiencing, especially the acidity buildup that had me relying on antacids for my own relief. I left the lecture motivated and went right to work planning meals that were compatible.
>
> At first it seemed difficult, but as I worked with it, I found it became easier. It was certainly worth the time and effort. The best part was how good I felt. All miserable symptoms were gone and for the first time in my life, I lost pounds without even trying. In fact, I dropped 10 pounds in two weeks.
>
> I have a 25-year-old daughter who has been suffering with severe bloating and gas pains after her meals. I have taken her to several doctors who were not able to help her, so I called her to try Proper Food Combining.
>
> She called me three days later, thrilled to tears because of her immediate results. She told me it was the first time in years that she didn't have to leave the table after dinner to unzip her pants or dress. She also dropped weight immediately without actually dieting.

Here's a letter from a woman who was on my

herbs and was *not* using Proper Food Combining:

> The first five days was quite a surprise after being on and trying so many programs. I've even gone on juice fasts which I thought were great. But the herbal formula does a thorough cleansing job. The sixth day on it, I found hard, black stones the size of a nickel or more, that looked like Apache tear stones. The eighth day, many, many deposits like large cucumber seeds. The eleventh day on for three months, there was residue coming out like chewed tobacco along with 18-inch or larger braid-like strings about the thickness of a nickel.

> After 4½ months, I'm still finding many strange things being expelled. I've had some cramping — remember we talked about it — but feeling so much better after losing a total of 24½ pounds with 14½ inches total loss over my whole body.

> My mental being or thinking is so much better. I used to eliminate once a day but never felt like it was complete. After the second week, I was eliminating six times a day. (Now we know where those extra meals have been.) And now I eliminate three to four times per day. I was wearing size 18 slacks and I now wear size 12. I cannot say enough about your herbal cleansing program. It's the best.

This letter is from a woman in her 60s.

> I love to wear my clothes and feel all that extra material I don't need anymore.

> I love to go to bed and know I will wake up in the morning without experienc-

ing that bad stomach I used to have.

I love the good taste in my mouth and all the juices that surge through it. It was always so dry and foul tasting before.

I love to make our meals and eat them — everything tastes so good now.

My family tells me I am so much more calm and not so nervous; — which is nice to hear.

I can keep going all day now and get a lot of things accomplished.

Every day is an exciting adventure and I look forward to feeling even better as I have been on this program only five months and still have a lot of cleansing to do.

I got George back on the program too. Much easier for me now!

I mentioned one person who had lost 25 pounds in five days. The same girl had lost 100 pounds under a doctor's care a year previously, but she was very gaunt-looking. She had lost all her breast tissue, but she still had her hips and thighs, so she purposely gained the weight back because she looked so out of proportion from her waist down.

When she went on my program, she lost 120 pounds in three months. She was not flabby; she did not lose even a half inch from her breasts, but lost over 11 inches from her hips. Her poisons were in her hips and thighs, and that's where she lost the weight.

I've had many people send in a letter stating that they no longer have migraine headaches caused by toxic backup.

One woman has been on my program for five years. The difference in her skin tissue is so startling that people who have not seen her for a long time think that she has had a face lift. The woman is approximately 60 years old.

Lee's comment: Please note the chain reaction this person is experiencing throughout her whole body. The cleansing and proper feeding is helping the body eliminate various symptoms.

> I went from size 16 to size 12 after the first week of using the herbal formula and the food combining. Last year I lost weight on another system, but gained it all back. I weigh 150 pounds and want to reach 130.
>
> I have quit using the chlorpheniramine for my sinusitus. I still use the theodur for asthma, but have cut back to one tablet per day most of the time. I hope to be rid of the asthma eventually, as well as the allergies.
>
> I lost inches very fast and reduced the aching joints throughout my body. I still have the cellulite symptoms in the thighs, stomach and buttocks.
>
> I have much less discomfort in my colon. The inflamation must have been keeping me awake nights because I am sleeping much better now.
>
> Thank you again, Lee. Please keep up your wonderful life's work!

As noted above, these results are not unusual. In fact, they are very typical of the hundreds of letters we receive each year from clients around the world.

If you have some experience with my herbal formula and Proper Food Combining you'd like to share, please write to me at:

Lee DuBelle
P.O. Box 35860
Phoenix, Arizona 85069
(602) 863-2715

For information to obtain any products mentioned in this book, write or call for closest distributor.

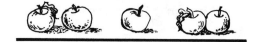

Other Information
and Resources
from Lee DuBelle

Proper Food Combining Cookbook: This cookbook contains many mouth-watering recipes, applying the basic principles of Proper Food Combining. It also includes a two-week menu guide. Spiral bound for easy use in the kitchen. (216 pages).

Internal Cleansing is an Old Movement: Learn ways to eliminate the toxins that have built up in your body over the years in order to restore the functions of your vital organs. This soft-bound book provides step-by-step instructions, as well as case studies (120 pages).

Combinando Correctamente Los Alimentos Funciona: This is the spanish translation of *Proper Food Combining Works*, produced especially for those whose first language is Spanish. (120 pages).

Proper Food Combining Charts: These laminated charts are produced in color and are invaluable for anyone interested in Proper Food Combining. They are available in two sizes: *Medium* (12"x9" folds to 6"x9") – can be slipped into book or tape album; and *Small* (6"x3.5" folds to 2"x3.5") – business card size, so that you can carry your food combining information with you.

Lee DuBelle's Cassette Tape Albums:

Series One: *"Proper Food Combining/Gaining Health, Losing Weight"* introduces Proper Food Combining techniques in a clear, easy-to-understand way, and discusses obesity as a disease that must be treated to produce increased health and well-being.

Series Two: *"Cleansing vs. Surgery"* demonstrates that cleansing organs is far superior to removal of them. It teaches the function and purpose of each organ and its importance to the body's operation and immune system.

Series Three: *"The Pre-Menstrual Syndrome/ Cellulite Connection"* discusses the interrelationships of PMS, menopause, hormones, cellulite, as well as how the endocrine system works.

Series Four: *"AIDS, Yeast Infection and Other Immune Diseases"* explores how the immune system works and what you can do to help the body build, or rebuild, its own immune system to prevent illness.

Lee DuBelle's Exercise Video: This 30-minute video teaches Lee's own personal exercise program utilizing gentle physical exercises and mild aerobics in conjunction with a slant board and mini-trampoline. the workout program is designed to tone the body's muscles and tissues to improve the operation of prolapsed organs and the immune system.

Proper Food Combining Video: This exciting and informative 70-minute video explains in detail how Proper Food Combining works. Learn to use the food combining chart, to recognize foods of each category, and to prepare easy recipes.

Colon Therapy Video: Lee made this 30-minute video with muscle therapist, Ron Geschwentner, to help you learn self colon therapy techniques. A valuable resource for anyone suffering from constipation, diarrhea, gas, diverticulitis or prolapsed colon, it includes laminated instructions for internal washing (enema).

LEEWEIGH DIET Cassette Tape Album: Finally a diet that builds health while you reach your desired weight and size. A diet according to the "body's design". A diet for *permanent* weight control. You've tried all the ones that don't work – now try the one that DOES!! Complete hour-by-hour menu and instructions.

ORDER FORM
Lee DuBelle
P.O. Box 35860
Phoenix, Arizona 85069
(602) 863-2715

QUAN.	DESCRIPTION	PRICE	TOTAL
_____	copies of *Proper Food Combining Works: Living Testimony*	$12.00	_____
_____	copies of *Combinando Correctamente Los Alimentos Fonciona*	$9.00	_____
_____	copies of *Proper Food Combining Cookbook*	$20.00	_____
_____	copies of *Internal Cleansing is an Old Movement*	$12.00	_____
_____	copies of laminated food combining chart		
	Medium (12 x 9 folds to 6 x 9)	$5.00	_____
	Small (folds to business card size)	$3.00	_____
_____	copies of audio cassette album #1 (4 tapes/6 hours) "Proper Food Combining/Gaining Health, Losing Weight"	$40.00	_____
_____	copies of audio cassette album #2 (4 tapes/4 hours) "Cleansing vs. Surgery"	$40.00	_____
_____	copies of audio cassette album #3 (4 tapes/6 hours) "The Pre-Menstrual Syndrome/Cellulite Connection"	$40.00	_____
_____	copies of audio cassette album #4 (4 tapes/3 hours) "AIDS, Yeast Infection, and Other Immune Diseases"	$40.00	_____

Total this page   _____

(continues on next page)

_____ copies of audio cassette album

(2 tapes/90 minutes) "LEEWEIGH
Diet" $25.00   _____
_____ copies of Exercise Video.
(30 minutes).VHS $30.00   _____
_____ copies of Proper Food Combining
Video. (70 minutes).VHS $50.00   _____
_____ copies of Colon Therapy Video.
(30 minutes). VHS $30.00   _____

Total from previous page   _____
Sub-Total   _____
Add shipping and handling – $5.00 first item,
75¢ each additional item
Canada: add $6.50 to above total   _____
Arizonans, please add 7.2% sales tax   _____
US FUNDS ONLY
TOTAL DUE   _____

Charge Card #_____

Exp. Date_____

Name _____

Address_____

City _____ State _____ Zip _____

Phone Number_____

❑   Please send more order forms.

❑   Please send free information packet.

ORDER FORM
Lee DuBelle
P.O. Box 35860
Phoenix, Arizona 85069
(602) 863-2715

QUAN.	DESCRIPTION	PRICE	TOTAL
_____	copies of *Proper Food Combining Works: Living Testimony*	$12.00	_____
_____	copies of *Combinando Correcta-mente Los Alimentos Fonciona*	$9.00	_____
_____	copies of *Proper Food Combining Cookbook*	$20.00	_____
_____	copies of *Internal Cleansing is an Old Movement*	$12.00	_____
_____	copies of laminated food combining chart		
	Medium (12 x 9 folds to 6 x 9)	$5.00	_____
	Small (folds to business card size)	$3.00	_____
_____	copies of audio cassette album #1 (4 tapes/6 hours) "Proper Food Combining/Gaining Health, Losing Weight"	$40.00	_____
_____	copies of audio cassette album #2 (4 tapes/4 hours) "Cleansing vs. Surgery"	$40.00	_____
_____	copies of audio cassette album #3 (4 tapes/6 hours) "The Pre-Menstrual Syndrome/Cellulite Connection"	$40.00	_____
_____	copies of audio cassette album #4 (4 tapes/3 hours) "AIDS, Yeast Infection, and Other Immune Diseases"	$40.00	_____

Total this page   _____

(continues on next page)

_____ copies of audio cassette album

(2 tapes/90 minutes) "LEEWEIGH
Diet" $25.00   _____
_____ copies of Exercise Video.
(30 minutes).VHS $30.00   _____
_____ copies of Proper Food Combining
Video. (70 minutes).VHS $50.00   _____
_____ copies of Colon Therapy Video.
(30 minutes). VHS $30.00   _____

Total from previous page   _____
Sub-Total   _____
Add shipping and handling – $5.00 first item,
75¢ each additional item
Canada: add $6.50 to above total   _____
Arizonans, please add 7.2% sales tax   _____
US FUNDS ONLY
TOTAL DUE   _____

Charge Card #_____

Exp. Date_____

Name _____

Address_____

City _____ State _____ Zip _____

Phone Number_____

❑   Please send more order forms.

❑   Please send free information packet.

ORDER FORM
Lee DuBelle
P.O. Box 35860
Phoenix, Arizona 85069
(602) 863-2715

QUAN.	DESCRIPTION	PRICE	TOTAL
_____	copies of *Proper Food Combining Works: Living Testimony*	$12.00	_____
_____	copies of *Combinando Correctamente Los Alimentos Fonciona*	$9.00	_____
_____	copies of *Proper Food Combining Cookbook*	$20.00	_____
_____	copies of *Internal Cleansing is an Old Movement*	$12.00	_____
_____	copies of laminated food combining chart		
	Medium (12 x 9 folds to 6 x 9)	$5.00	_____
	Small (folds to business card size)	$3.00	_____
_____	copies of audio cassette album #1 (4 tapes/6 hours) "Proper Food Combining/Gaining Health, Losing Weight"	$40.00	_____
_____	copies of audio cassette album #2 (4 tapes/4 hours) "Cleansing vs. Surgery"	$40.00	_____
_____	copies of audio cassette album #3 (4 tapes/6 hours) "The Pre-Menstrual Syndrome/Cellulite Connection"	$40.00	_____
_____	copies of audio cassette album #4 (4 tapes/3 hours) "AIDS, Yeast Infection, and Other Immune Diseases"	$40.00	_____

Total this page   _____

(continues on next page)

_____ copies of audio cassette album

(2 tapes/90 minutes) "LEEWEIGH
Diet" $25.00   _____

_____ copies of Exercise Video.
(30 minutes).VHS $30.00   _____

_____ copies of Proper Food Combining
Video. (70 minutes).VHS $50.00   _____

_____ copies of Colon Therapy Video.
(30 minutes). VHS $30.00   _____

Total from previous page   _____

Sub-Total   _____

Add shipping and handling – $5.00 first item,

75¢ each additional item

Canada: add $6.50 to above total   _____

Arizonans, please add 7.2% sales tax _____

US FUNDS ONLY

TOTAL DUE   _____

Charge Card #_____

    Exp. Date_____

Name _____

Address_____

City _____ State _____ Zip _____

Phone Number_____

❏   Please send more order forms.

❏   Please send free information packet.